HOW TO...
MOVE IT

How To... Move It

RESET YOUR BODY

JOSLYN THOMPSON RULE

1 3 5 7 9 10 8 6 4 2

#Merky Books

20 Vauxhall Bridge Road

London SW1V 2SA

#Merky Books is part of the Penguin Random House group of companies
whose addresses can be found at global.
penguinrandomhouse.com.

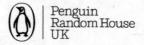

Copyright © Joslyn Thompson Rule 2021

Joslyn Thompson Rule has asserted her right to be identified as the author of this
Work in accordance with the Copyright, Designs and Patents Act 1988.

First published in the United Kingdom by #Merky Books in 2021

www.penguin.co.uk

A CIP catalogue record for this book is available from the British Library.

ISBN 9781529118902

Illustrations by Mica Murphy

Text Design © Andreas Brooks

Typeset in 10/13 pt Source Serif Variable Roman by Jouve (UK), Milton Keynes

Printed and bound in Great Britain by Clays Ltd, Elcograf S.p.A.

The authorised representative in the EEA is Penguin Random House Ireland,
Morrison Chambers, 32 Nassau Street, Dublin D02 YH68

Penguin Random House is committed to a sustainable future for our
business, our readers and our planet. This book is made from
Forest Stewardship Council® certified paper.

To BJ, Bjorn and Max - my three Kings

CONTENTS

FOREWORD

The concept of *how to move it* resonates with me so much because it's all I've ever known – from the bow-legged baby who learned to walk at seven months, playing the game of 'how quickly can I escape my mother?', to the 23-year-old Physiotherapy student who had a stroke and was diagnosed with multiple sclerosis, then decided she was going to do everything in her power to get back into sport, and eventually become a Paralympic champion and world record holder on the track and in the velodrome. Movement is the basis of everything we do, and the freedom to move is a luxury we sometimes take for granted.

Growing up, sport was a huge part of my life. I was *that* girl. The one who was annoyingly good at every sport and who you'd pick first to be on your team in PE. I played and participated in every sporting activity there was. Nothing was off limits. By the age of 21, I'd spent ten years as a dancer, seven years as a hockey player and ten years as an athletics sprinter, all with some overlap. I was Yorkshire and Northern champion in athletics, a medallist at national championships, inter-county competitions and British University champs, and my dance troupe had won the Leeds West Indian Carnival prize. Alongside my three main sports of dance, hockey and athletics, I enjoyed trampolining, gymnastics, football, netball, plus any other sport I could squeeze into my packed schedule. And boy was it packed! My secondary-school hockey coach used to drive me to the bus stop after a match so I could get to my athletics training on time. It was a hectic schedule, but my mother supported my passion, acting as my personal cheerleader and at times my personal chauffeur too. I wanted to do so much more, and really felt as if I could, as the freedom to move and be active is what I lived for.

So, in May 2014 when I woke up, barely able to move the right side of my body and unable to speak without slurring my words, my whole world came crumbling down. Movement, being active, playing sport – the things I loved and lived for – were taken away from me just like that. At the time of my stroke, I was in the first year of my Physiotherapy degree at Manchester Metropolitan University and knew that our motor system – part of the central nervous system – was a critical part of our movement, as all movement is created by nerve signals. To even begin to recover, I knew I had to create a new relationship with movement. So, I took it back to seven-month-old Kadeena – eager and determined to move – and used that memory as my driving force forward, one step at a time. It started with smaller actions, and smaller goals – from holding a fork to eat, or transferring my body out of my bed to a chair. These things were so big to me now, and losing the ability to do them seamlessly reminded me how much I loved the intricacies of the human body, how much freedom movement gives, and that I had something to fight for.

Then, just four months after my first stroke, I fell ill again. I woke up unable to move any of my limbs properly, I couldn't walk without support and I was in agonising pain. It was then that I was diagnosed with multiple sclerosis – a chronic illness (meaning a lifelong condition) that can severely affect your brain and spinal cord, and impair your vision, arm and leg movement, sensation in your body, and balance. This time was most devastating. I was housebound for three months. I lost my independence. I lost all the gains I had made. I lost the ability to care for myself. I lost my motivation.

During that time, my amazing mother was by my side and she stepped in to care for me, helping me wash and dress and making my meals.

My mother grew up in Jamaica, in a town called Rock Spring, in St Mary. Near her house there was a little stream that she used to run to, to bathe and wash her clothes. She was raised by her grandparents until she was a teenager and then came to live in Leeds with her mother, who had braved the journey to the UK on her own to start a new life. She has always been a vision of strength and independence for me, and the best role model I could have asked for. During this period, I drew on her tenacity as well as the strength I've witnessed first-hand through the generations of my family – from the ones who worked on the sugar cane fields in Jamaica, all the way down to my mother and aunts who are all nurses. Their dedication to keep pushing on – always with a smile on their face, may I add – combined with my faith in God is where my strength rose from in those very tough times.

The beauty of movement is that there is no set way. You just have to find your *why*. Everyone's *how* and *why* are different. Prior to getting ill, my *why* was purely that I loved sport and I wanted to see how far

I could push my body, unlocking its true potential. My current *why* is to show others that a lifelong health condition does not have to be a dead end; you can still enjoy your life and push yourself to achieve things even if they're done differently to how they used to be. I've always strived for perfection – it's in my nature as an elite athlete – and my diagnosis didn't stop my aspiration, it just changed the course of it a little bit. Your movement goal may be wanting to keep up with your children or grandchildren, to go for a kick-around in the park with your friends, or to do a morning yoga class. Whatever it is you want to do, you first have to appreciate how beautiful and how different our bodies are, and embrace every inch of that.

My journey of diagnosis, to recovery, to becoming a champion took hard work, a lot of tears and dedication. There were some highs and some lows, some victories and a lot of stumbles along the way, but I got there. We should all have goals, and be open to how they may change from time to time. But whatever your goal is, make sure you're enjoying it! That's what life is for. I'll admit I hate a lot of my training sessions at the time, but afterwards, the feeling of accomplishment that races through me is the ultimate satisfaction. Think about the smile that will stretch across your face after you finish your race, or lift that weight, or nail that yoga pose. That smile is what you'll remember and it can inspire someone else's day too.

My story may be very different to yours. With all my achievements – the first person in 32 years to win two gold medals in two different sports at the Paralympic Games, as well as setting a new world record on the athletics track and in the velodrome, five World Championship gold medals and being a Team GB flag-bearer at the 2016 Rio Olympics – I want to create a legacy for people with chronic illnesses and different movement abilities. I implore you to see the beauty in the freedom of movement. Take advantage of it, challenge yourself, and when things get tough, dig a little deeper because you will find something in you that you never realised you had. And if you've never seen someone like you do it before – it doesn't mean it can't be done.

– Kadeena Cox, MBE

INTRODUCTION

If you've picked up this book it means you want to start moving more; start moving better; or just want to try something different. I'm a fan of the basics, life is already complex. A better understanding of the basics, means better decision making for you, your body and your health. If everything you read here is new, that's great; if you know some stuff but other pieces of the puzzle connect for you, that's also pretty cool. Movement doesn't have to be complicated, you're already doing more than you think.

It's fair to say, I have an obsession with the process of change – no matter how big or small, it always starts with the mind. However, it's not what immediately comes to mind when people think of movement or sport, and why would it? The immediate thought is usually on the action/doing part, rather than the thinking part. Yet one doesn't exist without the other, and as you start on your journey of movement, my goal is to give you a good grasp of both to support you as best I can.

BROKEN DREAMS

I was born in Dublin in Ireland in 1978. I was the second eldest of four siblings – an older brother and two younger sisters. My mum worked in social services and my dad was a carpenter. When I was seven years old, he moved to England ahead of us to try and build a better life for our family. He came back for us six months later with a big lorry to move all our stuff to England. I remember begging my mum to let me go with my dad and brother to do one last trip to see a neighbour who we were giving our washing machine to. It was late at night and I should have been in bed, but I begged and begged. To stop my incessant whining, my mum gave in and let me go. When we returned, my dad decided to back the lorry into our driveway ready for the next morning. My brother stood behind the lorry and guided him in from the rear whilst I played around on the garden wall. As my dad reversed in, the side of the lorry got stuck on the gate attached to the wall I was standing on. 'The wall is wobbling!' my brother shouted at me. In my head I decided that walls don't wobble and carried on until the movement threw me off. The wall collapsed and landed on my left foot. Needless to say, I woke the entire neighbourhood with my cries. I'm pretty sure we ran every red light to get to the hospital.

I'd broken my foot and would need nine operations to fix it, including the amputation of my left big toe. After my last operation, the surgeon sat me on his knee and told me I would never be able to Irish dance again. I had danced and competed since the age of four. I loved it and even had a trophy or two under my belt. I remember blocking out what he said and deciding there and then that I would dance again – not in an 'I'll-show-you' kind of way, but because I wanted to dance, so I would. My resoluteness has stayed with me into adulthood. I'm often asked, 'What would you tell your younger self?', but there's not really anything I have to tell her: she still guides me! I'm not sure where she got her can-do attitude from, but she never asked for permission, ever, and she saw no limitation in being different. As adults, it's harder to see through the odds you stack up against yourself. Nevertheless, no matter what advice I'm given about barriers to overcome, my seven-year-old defiance, wrapped in curiosity, just wants to check if it's a definite 'No' before moving on.

BECOMING SOMEONE THROUGH SPORT

In 1997, after twelve years' living in England, I went back to Dublin to study at Trinity College. Dublin had definitely changed as a city since I'd lived there in the eighties; there were more people of colour than I remembered growing up. Now, I felt the difference of class. My parents were working class – after we left our family home in 1994, my mum worked as a cleaner in Tottenham to make ends meet and we grew up knowing the value of money. Yet here I was at a well-to-do university, surrounded by students with private school educations and money. I never felt more out of my depth. By accident, I took up rowing – and found that I was pretty good at it. I didn't have the height for a rower, but I was stronger than I looked and my technique was good – down to my Jamaican rhythm, apparently.

Soon after I started rowing, other students started to admire my athleticism; rowing was tough, which meant I was too. I was starting to feel like I was someone in these rich parts. I still had my part-time jobs and daydreamed about coming from a family that had money, but I also realised two important things: one, I didn't have much, but I was worth something, and two, nobody could take this strength away from me. I owned it, and that felt fucking good. Looking back now, I'd never have wanted this journey to be any other way.

Three years into my four-year economics degree, I became Vice Captain of the Ladies Boat Club at Trinity College. Little me from Tottenham. As Vice

Captain, I coached the novices alongside the Head Coach, Jonny. Jonny was ace; he really cared about us, like a coach should. He gave his heart and soul to our crew and I'm not sure we ever appreciated it at the time. I do now.

That year, coaching the novices taught me what it was like to take someone from a complete beginner to a rower who was able to shift the boat with power. I loved it and remember feeling beyond proud of their achievements. I may have had a different background to them, but I realised that we were all fighting our own battles, which disappeared, if only for a moment, with the sweet hypnotic sound of the oars lifting out of the water in unison. I also learnt fairly early on that whilst rowing is exceptionally physical, the mental demands are much greater. Understanding this became key to my coaching style (but more on that in the next chapter).

BECOMING A COACH

The amazing experience I had coaching at uni led me to decide that I wanted a career in fitness. After university, I spent a year teaching English in Japan, then returned to the UK to complete my Personal Training and Sports Therapy diploma in 2003. At that time, social media was in its infancy and a personal trainer profile was a picture of yourself and a short bio describing who you were and what you did, placed in the foyer of your local gym. Things have definitely changed since then. I lucked out starting at the time I did, when you could focus on your craft – and social media was not in the background making you question who you were, what you did and how you looked. I was able to just get my head down and learn from really good coaches around me, and I am thankful for that to this day.

Early on in my career, I became really interested in injury rehabilitation. I assisted football physios for a couple of seasons and that taught me a lot. To see people have a newfound appreciation for their body having gone through the disciplined process of physical rehabilitation never gets old for me. Physical rehab takes time, consistency and unbreakable trust in the process. It's also a magnifying glass on how our bodies readily compensate for weaknesses to allow us to keep going – until we get injured, that is.

SPORT CHANGES LIVES

Seven years into my career as a personal trainer, I was signed by Nike to be one of their Master Trainers.

This involved a long interview process to ensure my values were aligned with theirs, which are: 'do the right thing', 'be on the offense always', 'serve athletes', 'create the future of sport', and 'win as a team'; they are still aligned to this day. If you look up the 'If you let me play' video they made in 1995, you will understand the connection I have to the brand – I still get emotional watching it. I'm so grateful to have travelled around the globe delivering trainer education and training sessions, working on global campaigns – both behind and in front of the camera – and being part of some magical events bringing movement to people for the first time. For example, in 2015, 10,000 women ran the Nike 10k in London, a large percentage of whom were new to training; it's these journeys that make my work worth it.

Of all the incredible jobs I've done, one shows above all others how much sport and movement can transform and enhance your life. I was part of the Nike Training Club (NTC) initiative, which at the time was a comprehensive training programme for women (it is now dual gender), covering strength, endurance, yoga and mobility through both live classes and the NTC app. We took this programme into schools and tailored it to fifteen- and sixteen-year-old girls. My job was to deliver the training to twenty students, dubbed the 'naughty' girls of the year. Their PE teacher would shadow me for this session, and then run them alone after that. I had done countless sessions like this before, but I took extra time to prepare my music so the girls would think I was cool. Five minutes into the session a chorus of 'My make-up's running', 'My legs hurt' and 'I can't, Miss' ensued. We made it through the rest of the class, just, and I wished the teacher the best of luck as I left, thinking, 'They are never doing this class again.' Fitness isn't for everyone and that's OK.

Six weeks later, I returned to the school for their sports week. I sheepishly went over to the PE teacher and asked her how the sessions were going. She beamed with enthusiasm, telling me that two of the students led ten minutes of the class each week; they had changed their timetables so that they could all train first thing on a Friday morning (so there were no more make-up-running woes); they had encouraged the younger years to join them; and that they had kicked off the school sports day with a 5km run. I couldn't believe it. What I felt when I started rowing had happened to them. They had realised their bodies were strong and capable, and that gave them an inner strength and confidence that nobody could take away from them. I wrote them all a letter of appreciation as it felt like it had changed my life more than it had changed theirs – to my shame, I had already decided that this training thing wasn't going to work out for them. They showed *me* the transformational power of sport and that I should not have given up on them, they were only getting started.

SPORTY DOESN'T MEAN SPORT

The dread of 'sport' in our early years can create negative associations that stick with us forever. But let's just check in on those thoughts. When you say you were never good at sports in school – is that actually true, or was it a particular sport that wasn't for you? Maybe it was that sport, not all sport. You might think, 'But Joslyn, the thought of entering the gym still fills me with dread!' or 'I just don't feel sporty enough.' At Nike we have a saying: 'If you have a body, you're an athlete.' Fitness marketing feeds the stereotype of what 'sporty' looks like. The irony is that if you look across the spectrum of sports – from long-distance runners through to shot putters, the clients I train and all the bodies in between – there isn't just one look. Yet the six-pack body still reigns supreme, and we instinctively think that because I don't look like that, I'm not sporty. Let me repeat this one more time – if you have a body, you're an athlete.

CELEBRATE EVERY BODY

I've worked with some incredible elite athletes, but there is something special about working with regular people – and seeing how seemingly small changes in movement make a huge impact on a person's life – that makes my job so rewarding. One of my most memorable clients was a man in his fifties. Work and life had taken its toll on him physically and mentally, so we worked on him getting to feel more like himself through training. After six months of working together, he said to me, 'This will mean nothing to you, Joslyn, but I can tie my shoelaces for the first time in ten years.' Mean nothing? That meant everything to me! It still makes me proud when I think about it. Professional athletes have a team of people around them making them great. This guy did the work himself and his life changed as a result. I believe that journey of self-discovery is there for everyone, and every body.

FOR THE GRAM

I've briefly mentioned the pressure that social media can place on you, and how grateful I was to come up the ranks before it was so all-consuming – but I'm not going to hate on it entirely. Because of it, I've met some really good friends, reconnected with old school friends, and it's been a great tool for my line of work. However, I do recognise that it can be damaging beyond belief.

When it comes to fitness, social media is incredibly ableist. The word 'perfect' in conjunction with the word 'body' epitomises what it means to be fit. It affects those wanting to take their first step towards what healthier means for them; and it makes wannabe fitness professionals question whether or not they 'look' like a trainer. I know some incredible coaches who are held back from doing their best work because they feel like they don't fit the mould. Some of the most respected coaches I know are far from bearing a six pack. Their knowledge is their power, and their bodies have no bearing on the power they help to guide in others.

So much of the marketing in the fitness industry takes our power and control over our bodies away, telling us we need this diet or this training method to get results fast. Except our bodies are phenomenal machines, more complex and intelligent than any system or technology. If we start to understand our true power, that relentless marketing starts to weaken – we start looking within for what we can do, instead of passing our hopes for our bodies to another person, diet or exercise system.

FOR YOU

If there is one thing I want you to take away from this book, it's that you are the most important person in your life. This may sound harsh, but nobody is coming to save you; your focus on moving forward has to be coupled with your focus on looking within – it's a decision for you, from you. I'm a personal trainer, people come to me for guidance, but they do the work. One of the final questions I ask in an initial client consultation is: 'What do you think *you* need to do?' If I just take their money and tell them what to do, then I am perpetuating the message from marketing that 'You need me, so I can fix you!' It's the opposite. As a personal trainer I am here to guide you, and what I need to know is how invested you are in this, not just financially but emotionally.

WHAT THIS BOOK IS

Consider reading this book to be a fresh start in how you communicate with yourself around fitness. The fitness industry is very outcome-based: eat this, sweat lots, look this way. If the process of how to move it was a pyramid, for me mindset would be at the bottom, and the next layer would be sleep, breathing and general movement – the stuff we already do daily that we don't see as 'exercise', contributes a lot to our overall health. Quite frankly, the less sexy stuff is always more important, and understanding this means you've already made a start in changing your attitude towards movement.

This is why, before we get to the exercise, we start with the most important part of the body: the brain. The relationship you have with yourself is the most important relationship you will ever have – how you communicate with yourself is everything.

We then look at understanding the body better. We are complex, beautiful beings – our operating system is far superior to anything else that we know – but our default is not always the most efficient way to move and be.

Once we understand our inner workings, ever nurturing our mindset, we get to what we commonly know as movement: mobility, strength, cardiovascular fitness and recovery. You'll learn what it is, and how to incorporate it into your life – and, most importantly, how to have fun with it.

Lastly, this book inspires you to take it one step further. You'll be pointed in the direction of what to do next. Once you have a new view of what movement is, you can make it a part of your life, your way.

CHAPTER I

HEAD IN THE GAME

I'm obsessed with the organ where your thinking takes place. Did you know your brain weighs a mere 3lb? Yet it's more powerful than we realise; it can take a suffocating hold on us – or it can liberate us beyond belief. Psychological challenges overshadow physical ones in so many sports, and at the elite level, mental strength is what separates the top percentage of world athletes. But it's not just in sport that this matters; it applies to how we think, every single moment of every single day. If we learn to create awareness around a small percentage of our limiting beliefs, we are winning. Building mental strength is daily work, and can be more taxing than the physical effort, even if a little mundane! As a pro at getting those new to exercise started on a running journey, my friend Cory Wharton-Malcolm says, 'to get good at something, you have to master boredom'. Everyone's looking to *stay* motivated, because that's the secret, right? Sometimes the work is in just showing up repeatedly, even when your mind has other ideas.

Belief is everything and the hardest thing. At some point, you just have to decide – it's that simple. Sometimes it's easier to hide behind all the reasons you can't do something than to bravely make the decision that you can and then act on it. That elusive state of being 'in the zone' that we hear competitive athletes refer to is ours for the taking too, even if we're not on the world stage for a given sport. We have to remember that our bodies are incredible, and our minds control it all.

MIRACLES OF THE MIND

About seven years ago, I became really aware that I put too much focus on what others thought of how I trained. At the time I was competing in crossfit and local strong woman competitions and I didn't like the feeling of worrying so much about what others thought. I knew that giving so much energy to the opinions of others couldn't be good for me, and a friend recommended Katie Page, a sports psychologist who she thought could help me.

On our first call, Katie told me her story and I listened with my mouth open. When Katie was nineteen, she had been placed in the top three at Junior Nationals in horse eventing and was also hoping to compete for Great Britain in rowing. Then she suddenly fell ill with a rare neurological disorder, transverse myelitis (TM), which wound up paralysing her. She lost the full use of her arms and legs – and her dreams of rowing for Great Britain and eventing slipped away almost overnight. Katie would end up needing full-time care at a specialist facility.

At the end of the first day in the facility, Katie called her mother and told her she could not stay because she believed she wasn't going to get better there. Katie and I are poles apart in terms of the damaging effect of her condition and my experience of my own accident, but I connected with her hope. That seven-year-old and that nineteen-year-old decided something different about their 'fate'. We both refused to listen to the experts and listened instead to our own desires. Anybody with an opinion on your ability can stop you in your tracks – a parent, a doctor, a friend. A simple, 'I'm afraid you will not be able to [*insert your desire*] again', or worse, 'Are you sure you can do this?' are the words that get you doubting yourself. They sting because 'not doing it' never crossed your mind and now it's all that you can think of. 'Can I? Can I really do this?' you ask yourself.

I was in awe speaking to Katie. Refusing to sit in a wheelchair or lie in bed, Katie knew she still had her mind. 'Even when my body was dead, I was imagining it moving. I kept visualising myself being active.' Within a few days, and with the full use of her hands, Katie signed up for online tuition to train her mind, and to train her body to get better. Within four months of being diagnosed with an incurable condition, Katie could stand up from her wheelchair. Within nine months, she could walk again. After being told there was no way she could have children, she is now a mother of two. For Katie, there were many times when she believed that doctors were right about her not being able to have children, but she knew she had to do the focused mindset work to get there. And it was work. Consistent work. Katie's fight gives me faith in miracles of the mind. But once you have control of your mind, you still need to work on it, even if you are a mindset boss like Katie.

ACTIVE MINDSET

Katie was my first introduction to active mindset work. I remember relaying to her how tiring it was to really try and get a grip on my thoughts. I suddenly became so aware of the negative voice in my head, it felt relentless – 'You're just not good enough', 'Everyone else finds this easier than you' – but becoming aware of my thoughts was the first step. She told me it takes time to rewire our brains. Initially you aren't even aware of your negative thoughts, let alone able to do something about them; but then you start to notice them, and once you sense them coming, you can learn to nip them in the bud before they take hold.

SELF-TALK MATTERS

How you communicate with yourself is really bloody important. I need to be honest here; if this shit was easy, we'd all be fist pumping upon waking and breezing through the day. You're not expected to be positive all the time, that's not the point.

I remember when I had to learn to walk again, the most important conversations were those I had with myself. It started with being fully supported and just being upright. Getting used to that. Then some weight bearing. That ached, and that made a reality of the large mountain ahead. I cried and I wanted the aching to stop, because I couldn't dance if it was going to hurt like this. 'You can do this,' I coached myself, 'he is not going to stop you from dancing'. The surgeon was so kind to me – but in those moments I hated him: he was stopping my dreams, he had taken my toe away.

Soon enough the aching subsided and I was able to do more. With hands firmly gripping the parallel supports, I would tense my whole body as I lifted my right foot – my good foot – so that I was fully supported on my left. My whole body would shake and I would hold my breath, but as my right foot returned back to the ground, I realised I was doing it. I was walking. In my mind I mapped it out. One day I would walk without holding on, and tensing and wobbling. One day it would stop aching. Then I'd be dancing. Then it would be done.

This could have been different; I was told by others what I couldn't do, but I chose not to tell myself the same thing. No matter where you are starting from on your fitness journey, the voice that holds the most power, the voice that knows you the most, is your own.

THE SELF-TALK AUDIT

In the words of Mental Performance Coach Justin Su'a, what you need to do is stop listening to yourself and start talking to yourself. Fears will interrupt every moment of your day if you let them – a little voice of self-doubt sabotaging your efforts. In his book, *The War of Art*, Stephen Pressfield calls this voice 'resistance'. The closer you get to reaching your goals, the more pissed off 'resistance' gets and really tries to break up the party. Now you know that voice is a part of the process, but you don't have to give it power. You just need to know it's a persistent little fucker.

Let's examine how we talk to ourselves. This exercise will help you see just how negative our thoughts can be unless we get a hold on them.

STEP 1: Consider your goal

Think of a movement/fitness goal you already have. Don't overthink it. Got it? Good! Now what was your very next thought? I don't know you, but I'm guessing that it was something to the tune of 'you can't do that', 'that's so hard!', 'how do you think you are going to do that?'

STEP 2: Break down that negative thought

First, ask yourself, 'Is it true?' Do you have clear evidence that this thought is a reality? There's no 'ummm' here, it's a 'yes' or 'no' answer. And I'm going to guess that it's a 'no'.

STEP 3: Repeat

Let's try again. Think of a different goal. What's the very next thought? Is pesky persistence still there? It's not? OK, you're doing great! You've taken the first step. You've started to observe how you sabotage your own goals the second they enter your head, and are now making a conscious effort to stop it. Focus on what your next step is. Actually, ask yourself, 'What's my next step?', 'What can I do right now to make that happen?', 'Who can I ask for guidance?'

The self-talk audit is step one in rewiring our communication, and how we communicate with ourselves. Thick-skinned or not, right or wrong, receiving criticism is never easy in the moment. We're human and one of our biggest in-built desires is to belong. I'm a huge advocate of learning from failures, but it doesn't mean they don't suck at the time. And so if one of our biggest desires is to belong, then not belonging, being judged, is one of our greatest fears.

LANGUAGE TO SELL

Whilst we're on the subject of language, one of the things that sports advertising companies do really well is use big powerful language in their campaigns.

We're told to 'push', 'drive', 'power', 'sweat' or 'go hard or go home'. In reality, it's subtler than that: it's the phrases 'one step at a time', 'little and often' and 'consistency' that will have just as powerful an effect. I have two issues with the language often used by the sports companies.

ABILITY

What if I am not able to do any of these things? Is there a space for me in the world of health and fitness? Could my sports psychologist, Katie Page, have done any of those things when she lay quadriplegic in a hospital bed? What about one of my clients, Steve, who had myalgic encephalomyelitis (ME)? Are they sharing the message that there wouldn't be any point for him? We also have to think about the conditions we can't see – what if sweating is exactly what someone dealing with anxiety experiences every day? No thank you, ableism. A lot of assumptions are made around the starting point of 'being the best you', but where does that leave you if the starting point is not a place where you currently reside? You don't get to start? Sorry, it's just not for you? Movement is a privilege and requires more than just motivation so that we can all take part. We must do better.

REALITY

This message, and these adverts, paint a picture of a very small moment in time, and only apply to some sports. Yes of course there are times to push, drive, power, but that's largely driven by your mind and not your body. Go and look at a video of Usain Bolt before a race; the fastest man in the world shows no signs of these active words – he is calm, relaxed, ready to use every cell of his being to perform.

POSITIVE PRACTICES

I've said it more than once now, but I'll say it again. Getting your mind right is work – consistent work – but bloody well worth it, I promise you. But since we have a lot of negative thoughts floating around in our heads, it's pretty useful to tackle a little each day, to lighten the load.

Here are some methods that can help you to alleviate your mental stress.

MEDITATION: SLOW DOWN

I have tried lots of different types of meditation over the years, and what works best is what you need at that time. If you find it really difficult, go for a guided meditation. The Headspace app is an easy and simple go-to; even my five year old listens to the children's one. The meditation takes as little as 5–10 minutes a day, and if you haven't got 5–10 minutes to spare in all the minutes of the day, well . . . I have no words. You absolutely have 5 minutes, but I'm also down if you start with one or two!.

LAUGHTER: WORK YOUR FACE MUSCLES

A good nutritional therapist friend of mine absolutely hates the idea of meditation and recommends laughter instead. When my aunty was dying with pancreatic cancer, part of her therapy was laughter. Both her and my uncle would watch comedies together because laughter has such a positive effect on our physiology – the absolute opposite of the depressing things we see every day in the news! So, if meditation is really not your thing, then try a good stand-up show instead.

JOURNALING: GET IT ON THE PAGE

Get all of those thoughts out of your head and onto paper. There have been times when I have just written and written, until eventually that thing that was on my mind lightens. Sometimes I even find solutions, which is pretty dope.

SHOWER: STAND AND SOOTHE

I'm not suggesting you need a wash, but I always find that things come to me when I'm in the shower; I call them 'douche downloads'. It's a very simple activity and there's not much to do but to be still in your mind, then, splash! (sorry, very bad joke), a solution or thought comes out of nowhere that is really damn helpful.

All of these activities just create a little bandwidth for our minds so we can gain more clarity and get better at turning down the noise.

CHAPTER 2

THE PEP TALK

It's important to understand that we should never base our self-worth on the approval of others. Yes, friends, family and supportive coaches are all amazing and are sure to pick you up when you are down. But there is only one person who is with you every moment of every day: you! It makes sense then that you get to decide what it is you really desire on this fitness journey and set the path to get there, through understanding your why and setting intentions.

KNOW YOUR WHY

When I first meet new clients, they come in and tell me their goal. They can often be fairly generic, like, 'I want to get fit.' This is pretty vague. I have no doubt they want to get fit, but I want to know why they want to get fit? What impact will that have on their lives?

Getting clear on your 'why' is a tool I first learned from author and founder of Precision Nutrition, Dr John Berardi, who was influenced by a practice used by Toyota Motor Corporation to solve problems. The '5 Whys' analysis was originally developed by Sakichi Toyoda, and was used to trace the root cause of the problems within the manufacturing process of Toyota cars. Toyoda advocated that, when faced with a problem, the key is to ask 'Why?' five times to try and get to the root cause of the problem. For example: Why were you late for work? Because I missed my train. Why did you miss your train? Because I couldn't find my keys. Why couldn't you find your keys? Because I forgot I wore a different jacket yesterday and left them in it. What could prevent this from happening again? I could have a place for my keys at home so I always know where they are. Where will you leave them? On the hallway shelf. This same method can really help you to understand your goals. Let's start with a common example: 'I'm tired!'

WHY are you tired? Because I went to bed late last night.

WHY did you go to bed late last night? Because I had to finish a piece of work.

WHY didn't you finish it sooner? Because I was putting it off and watched a programme instead.

WHY did you put it off for so long? Because I didn't plan my time well enough.

WHY didn't you plan your time? Because I underestimated how long the task would take.

Questioning each previous answer helps to find a solution for what needs to be done. You would not necessarily associate being tired with not having planned your week out, but the two are very much connected. Now let's try a different example with the method – one that will help you understand the 'Why?' behind your movement goal: 'I want to get fit.'

WHY do you want to get fit? Because I feel tired all the time.

WHY do you feel tired all the time? Because simple things like taking the stairs leave me breathless.

WHY do you mind being breathless? Because it makes me feel self-conscious.

WHY do you mind feeling self-conscious? Because it increases my anxiety and I want to feel less anxious.

WHY do you want to feel less anxious? Because I want to be relaxed and enjoy the time I spend with my family and friends.

We often think we know what it is that we want, but it's not until we go deeper that we understand the true reasons behind why we want to do something.

However, if your 'Why?' is concerned with how you look and wanting to lose weight, make sure you are doing it for you, not anybody else. You can absolutely do what you want with your body; don't be shamed into losing weight because of what [insert person(s) name who has no bearing on your life] wants you to look like based on their own experience. Screw them; it's *your* body. If you want to lose weight for you, do it. If you don't want to lose weight for you, don't do it. When you make either of those decisions for somebody else, it's time to find out what *you* want, because that's the only thing that matters.

SET INTENTIONS

OK, let's recap a little. Have you been working on the mindset stuff I talked about in the first chapter? Because if you think you can skim over that bit, I'm here to be the voice of reason – your thoughts are everything and they will control you if you don't build awareness around them. In fact, if you haven't done any of the exercises related to mindset just yet, stop reading right now and go back! You can't move until you become aware of your thoughts. If you have been working on them – well done!

Setting intentions for the day or week ahead is like giving your end goal a blessing. It's a loving hug from yourself to yourself. It's not something you force. The trick to intentions is the phrasing and words that you use. When you set an intention, apply a positive caveat to it rather than a negative one. Imagine your goal and think, 'If this thing happened today, that would be cool,' rather than, 'I have to do this today or else.' That has a whole different energy about it. Don't think for a second that I'm suggesting you float your way through life hoping for the best, but life can feel high pressure at the best of times, and an 'if' can just feel lighter than a 'should'.

Let's look at some examples. Let's say your goal is to get fit because you want to be relaxed and enjoy your time around your family and friends. Your intentions could be:

1. Today, if I find myself feeling anxious, I will pause and take three deep breaths.

2. Today, I will take 20 minutes out of my day to move my body, even if it's just to do some gentle stretching or mobility exercises.

3. Today, I will write down three things that I am grateful that my body can do.

None of these by themselves will get you to your goal, but they will all contribute to keeping you on the right track. They don't have to be the same every day – they are of your choosing with each new day. If you don't get to do one or all of them, that's OK too. They are intentions, not rules to live or die by, so simply try again tomorrow – maybe take just one deep breath, or move for 10 minutes, or write down one thing you're grateful for.

Set between one and three intentions for your day and reflect on them at the end of it.

REFRAME ALL OF IT

In chapter 1 we discussed negative thoughts and questioning whether they are true or not as a first port of call. But it doesn't stop them coming – they are relentless. Some thoughts come back again and again, no matter how much you are aware of them and try to rationalise them. When this happens, you can reframe how you see things. Rather than telling yourself the negative, try spinning that thought to see it from the positive. So when that limiting thought slips in just before you're about to go for your run, it's time for a reframe.

ORIGINAL THOUGHT: 'I'll never be able to run a mile.'

REFRAME: 'With each training session, I am one step closer to running a mile.'

ORIGINAL THOUGHT: 'I'll never be good enough.'

REFRAME: 'I am doing the best I can with the resources I have now, and I continue to work on building my skills.'

ORIGINAL THOUGHT: 'While I am half of two things, I'll never feel whole.'

REFRAME: 'I am whole, I'm just a special blend.'

'I'll never' (future-focused) becomes 'I am' (in the present). All you have absolute control over is what you are doing now in the present moment. Small steps repeated over time make big changes, but you must stay focused on where you are now, especially when where you want to get to seems so far away. You still have to get there the same way, taking a step in each moment and keeping your focus there.

> Write down the negative thoughts that keep coming back for you.
>
> Now reframe them. How does that change in belief feel?

After you have mastered reframing all those negative beliefs, it can be fun to say 'Screw you' whenever they try to take over. It's empowering to know you have the ability to re-evaluate those limiting beliefs, rather than giving in to them.

MENTAL IMAGERY

After about a month or so of working with Katie Page, she introduced me to the idea of mental imagery – seeing something in your mind's eye. She explained to me that when you imagine something, your brain believes that it is really happening. I had heard of the concept before, but it took me a while to get my head around it!

Katie told me about the 'Piano study' from Harvard University, which compared the brains of people who actually played a sequence of notes on the piano and those who *imagined* playing the same sequence of notes for two hours a day, over five days. At the end of the five-day experiment, a brain scan was taken of both groups. The findings were extraordinary; the region of the brain which controls the muscles in the fingers had changed to the exact same degree in both groups of participants. Even though one group had actually practised on a piano and the other just imagined it, the brain could not tell the difference.

I gave it a try. There was a particular weight that I feared when doing a snatch – one of the Olympic weightlifting movements where you lift the barbell from the floor to overhead at speed. It requires you to start the lift with control, and then powerfully pull yourself underneath the bar as the weight is still travelling upwards. That's the part where I used to get a mental block. You want me to dive underneath that weight and hold it above my head in a squat position with my arms locked out? Gulps. I thought this might be a good place to start with mental imagery.

And so I started to visualise me powerfully pulling myself underneath the bar. I even had a song in my head to throw into the mix. I remember the snap of the beat being in my hips and the second I snatched it, it worked. Even my husband did a double take.

Now it's your turn. What video could you play out in your mind's eye that would move you closer to your fitness goal? Start simply, just a step or two ahead of where you are now as it will be easier to visualise it. Are you finishing a short run? Holding a plank for a certain time? Moving your body with energy and ease?

Imagine a future you. Where are you? What are you wearing? What can you see? What can you hear? What can you smell? Get all your senses involved. What are you doing? How does it feel?

The key with all of this imagery stuff is that it doesn't have to be perfect. My mental performance specialist friend Emma Hackett taught me that if the first video in your mind doesn't feel good, that's OK. The first draft will usually need some work. As you start to play out the vision, and a negative thought creeps in, start again. You could also play out all scenarios in your head; actively asking, 'What would I do if this happened?' is different from your negative thoughts crashing the party uninvited.

THE PROBLEM WITH PERFECTION

Perfectionism is a form of procrastination. Nobody cares how perfect something is, except you. It's a self-protection mechanism: if you never put yourself out there, you will never leave yourself open to criticism. I know this because I was a perfectionist; I nodded proudly when someone first labelled me so. It tied in with the good girl archetype of people-pleasing – yet the last person that served was me. I now say I'm a recovering perfectionist, but secretly it's always there; you know that scene in *Avengers Assemble* when Bruce Banner turns around as he morphs into the Hulk and says, 'That's my secret, I'm always angry'? That's how I feel about being a perfectionist; I'm just able to control it now.

Parkinson's law states that the more time we have to do something, the longer it will take. I don't always get it right, but if I set myself a strict deadline, and ignore the voice in my head that says I need to research more, or check one more thing, or redo a certain bit, then I make good decisions rather than finding unnecessary solutions to something that is already good enough. If we understand that there is no such thing as perfect, then it makes sense not to strive for it. Every step of your fitness journey does not have to be 100% for it to work or for you to progress. For the perfectionists among you, 70–80% is good, just keep it moving.

THE FOUR-QUESTION REVIEW

One of the most useful things Katie taught me was the four-question review. When I was being extremely negative or concerned with what others thought of me, she would get me to ask myself the following four questions.

1. What went well?

2. What would I do differently?

3. How does this give me confidence?

4. How does this make me feel better prepared?

Asking the four questions forces you to find a positive, and actually contemplate the action you would do the next time round so that you could achieve a different outcome.

A crucial question in the set of four is the second one, 'What would you do differently?' Let's say you committed to training twice a week. The first session felt very new but you enjoyed it, but in the second session you felt self-conscious and unsure if you were doing anything right. Why was that the case? What would you do differently if you had the same experience again? Maybe you could have looked at the exercises ahead of the session; maybe you were rushing and not paying attention to your form. Looking back over it and asking yourself what you would do differently next time gives you your power back; you become solution-focused rather than thinking negatively about it.

BE YOUR OWN CHEERLEADER

OK, I'm not sure how to put this, but not everyone is going to be happy about you making fitness a part of your life. It's absolutely nothing to do with you – although it may feel that way. It's hard to think that the people who know and love you might not have your back as much as you thought. They will be well meaning, and it will seem to come from a good place. Actually, it will come from a shit place – but from their shit place, not yours. They may say things like, 'I'm just telling you for your own good' (that's a punch-worthy comment, if ever there was one). This is what I warn my clients about in our first consultation. Once we've talked through their goals, we've made a plan and we are ready to go, I break the news to them that they may not get the support they need from those closest to them.

Some people can't bring themselves to say a simple 'well done' when your success and effort has held up a reflection of themselves that they don't like – they have been talking about getting back into exercise for years, and here you are, actually doing it. How irritating. It has so little to do with you, and yet you feel like it does, no matter how much you rationalise that their jealousy is about them. We're not innocent of this ourselves. Ask yourself the uncomfortable question: 'Have I done the same?' We all have – we see someone else's progress and we want a little bit of it too.

It may not make sense to others why you are doing what you are doing and it shouldn't have to. Whilst it would be nice for them to see beyond themselves and become part of the go-you campaign, you have to be prepared for them not to be, and that is OK. You have got you, remember?

THE TOOLS TO YOUR OWN SUCCESS

Success is an inside job; we sometimes just need some help to get us there. If we base our success around the approval of others then we are doing ourselves a disservice. The tools I have mentioned in this chapter are your support team – they help you become clear on what you want, reframe negative thinking, and keep you moving forward. I'm an impatient person. I absolutely believe in the long game in training, life and business, but if I can find a hack to help me get there, I will! That's why I always come back to these exercises. Doing the actual work and seeing the change as you do is magical. A lot of the time, that can feel uncomfortable, but that is part of the work. Picking up this book, contemplating your first run, or putting your PE kit on for the first time in a long time – it can feel a little scary, right? But the more times you do shit that scares you, the better you get at doing shit that scares you.

CHAPTER 3

KNOW YOUR BODY BETTER

I can hear you: 'Joslyn, this book is about moving it and you haven't mentioned a single dumbbell yet. Where exactly are we going with this?' First of all, how assumptive of you – who says I am going to make you lift weights or run? Well, I may, but let's not jump to any conclusions – yet. I need to get you mentally ready for the time when it comes.

MORE THAN MOVEMENT

You know that exercise will have a positive effect on your mind and body, but not knowing where to start, feeling huge discomfort at the thought of it or just not being arsed, can mean that you are unapologetically anti-exercise and couldn't give two hoots about gaining the momentum or the motivation. We've all been there. It's OK, we *all* get it.

Well, I'm going to let you in on a little secret. Learning 'how to move it' is about so much more than movement. No, I haven't been leading you astray – the exercise part is at the very top of the pyramid I described in the beginning. I just spent two chapters focusing on the most important muscle in your body – your brain. (Yes, I know only a small part of your brain is actual muscle, but it sounds good.) *Moving* more will help you feel good, but *feeling* good will help you move. And the great news is that we are already doing stuff that will benefit both our bodies and minds; we are already on the right path.

EVERYDAY SUPERPOWERS

Let's look at the cool stuff you are already doing that impacts your health in a big way. I'm talking about sleep, breathing and how you move about day to day. These are all the big players, even if this is the very start of your journey – or in fact, even if you're a pro. If you're someone who sleeps, breathes and has a level of independence over your daily movement, then you have got this.

SLEEP, YOUR SILENT SUPERPOWER

Sleep is the foundation of good health. When you sleep, you are giving your tissues a chance to grow and repair; growth hormone, essential for growth and development, is released; immune function is boosted; and your brain is rested so you are able to be mentally alert and to focus upon waking. Having less than the recommended seven to nine hours of sleep per night in the short term will lead to tiredness, irritability and difficulty focusing. Over the long term, the consequences are more serious, putting you at risk of heart disease, diabetes, mood disorders, obesity and reduced life expectancy. It really is the magic pill to health and fitness.

You may have hoped said magic pill was a little sexier than me saying go to bed for at least seven to nine hours every night. Sleep isn't sexy. And the less you sleep, the more time you have to do stuff, right? It's in-keeping with the hustle-hard mentality society leads us to believe we all need. Yes, sleeping less creates more time, but it also makes us operate at a reduced quality. How many times has someone told you to 'sleep on it' ahead of making a big decision or if you are upset by something? More sleep helps us to make better decisions; we've been telling ourselves and each other to do it for years.

I'm the first one to put my hand up to a getting-things-done obsession that has often led me into the early hours of the morning, exhausted but with the feeling of being super productive buzzing around me. It was only recently that I ditched that habit. A late night for me is now 11pm, not 2am or 3am. In the process of writing this book, getting to bed at a decent hour was a huge motivator for me. When my little boys wake up between 6:30–7am and insist on morning wrestles, time is no longer my own, and I don't want it to be. I decided to wake up at 5am to have a little headspace, which meant I was in bed at a very decent hour.

FIVE TIPS FOR BETTER SLEEP

1. Don't drink caffeine in the afternoon or evening as it will make it more difficult for you to get to sleep and will affect the quality of it. Even better, give it up.

2. Don't eat just before bed. We will have better-quality sleep if our bodies are not trying to digest food.

3. Get rid of any blue light activity 30–60 minutes before bed (that's phones, laptops, TV) as the blue light supresses the secretion of melatonin, the hormone that regulates our sleep/wake cycle.

4. Make sure your bedroom isn't too warm – our body temperature naturally drops at night, so going to bed in a cool room will signal to your body that it's time for sleep.

5. Keep the room dark as even a small amount of light can disrupt your sleep. I'm a fan of silk eye masks as they leave you less panda-esque upon waking!

Don't expect to get this right straight away. I've just listed five things that could well be very big adjustments in your life. As you work to improve your sleep, maybe 'quality' alone is your first focus, then maybe you can look at the quantity. Seven to nine hours is what's recommended, but if you are currently getting five to six hours, maybe simply improving the quality of those hours using the tips above is a start. Baby steps.

DEEP BREATHS, YOUR REGULAR SUPERPOWER

Inhale . . . exhale . . . We do this without thinking about it. Whether we do it efficiently is another matter. In movement there are lots of different ways to breathe to assist the task at hand, but I want to focus on simple breathing techniques that can improve our overall health. When someone says, 'breathe', 'just breathe', or 'deep breaths' in a moment of panic, intuitively we know that doing so will bring a level of calm. Breathing is instinctive, we know it helps when we focus on it, and let's not forget its major role in keeping us alive. So what if we were a little more proactive about this thing that we just do without thinking. Again, not a gym, dumbbell or kettlebell in sight yet, just doing what we already do a little better. You just got healthier. This fitness stuff is actually easy, but we need to make sure we have solid foundations.

ON THE COUNT OF THREE . . .

Let's take a look at how you breathe right now. Get comfy, wherever you are; if you're reading this on the bus, it's cool, you don't have to lie down for the next three stops, just make sure you're sitting comfortably. Place one hand on your chest and one hand above your stomach. Follow the pattern of your breathing. Can you feel your chest expand? Can you feel your stomach expand? Or both? If it's hard to feel, take some deeper breaths. After a few breaths you should be able to determine where you feel it the most. If you feel it more in your chest, you are a shallow breather – and we need to get you breathing like you mean it! If you feel it in your stomach (it doesn't actually go into your stomach, but it's a simple landmark, instead of you trying to locate your lungs), that means you are taking that air deeper into your lungs, which encourages your body to shift into a more relaxed state.

BREATHING AND THE NERVOUS SYSTEM

Breathing and our autonomic nervous system are inextricably linked. The ANS is a control system that acts unconsciously and regulates bodily functions, such as the heart rate, digestion, breathing, etc. We don't have to think about these functions, they just happen. The ANS has two main divisions: the sympathetic nervous system (SNS) and the parasympathetic nervous system (PNS).

The **SYMPATHETIC** nervous system puts the body in a state of readiness to 'fight or flight' in response to any potential danger. This was really useful for us when the threat of a lion chasing us was real. Today, the lion has been replaced with everyday stressors like workload, exams, finances and the fast-paced demands of technology. There is no longer the peak of danger before you go back to not worrying about being eaten; these everyday stressors keep us in a heightened state of stress for a longer period of time, over relative low-level dangers. This consistently stressed state eventually impacts our health.

On the other hand, the **PARASYMPATHETIC** nervous system inhibits the body from overworking and restores it to a state of 'rest and digest', which allows us to recover adequately before we are demanded to be 'on' again. This used to happen naturally after running away from danger, but if we understand that modern living keeps us in this ongoing stressed state, it is important for us to try and bring ourselves out of the sympathetic state and into a restorative parasympathetic state. Focusing on our breathing can help us do this. The well-intentioned 'just breathe' can be even more beneficial when we know how to breathe fully.

DIAPHRAGMATIC BREATHING

The diaphragm is the primary muscle used in the process of breathing or respiration. It is located just below the heart and lungs, contracting as you inhale and relaxing as you exhale. Diaphragmatic breathing is a simple practice that expands your diaphragm to its full capacity, helping you use your lungs more efficiently. Mastering it will help you bring yourself down from that 'ready' state.

Get comfortable again, but now place your hands around your ribs. As you breathe in, think about expanding your ribs out to the sides. It's common to be told to breathe into your belly, but that's not our goal here; we want to experience a full 360-degree expansion of your torso – the back, the sides and the front, to reflect the full inhalation we are taking. This may feel a little weird at first, you may even feel a little dizzy: if you do, take a rest. Once you feel like you are getting that full 360 degrees of expansion, you are going to take several deep breaths – start at three with a goal to work up to ten over time:

1. Breathe in for a count of four.

2. Hold your breath for a count of two.

3. Exhale for a count of six.

Taking moments throughout the day to take three to ten deep breaths will make a big difference. I breathe like this when I wake up, I breathe like this before I train, and I breathe like this before I go to sleep.

It may seem odd to want to stimulate parasympathetic nervous system activity before you train, but before warming up to a state of readiness, you need to start from a place of calm. Once, an incredible coach and friend of mine was questioned about why she'd added breathing as a first exercise in her strength class. The well-meaning coach asserted that he 'wouldn't advise stimulating the parasympathetic nervous system before training . . .' He had failed to see the bigger picture in her planning. Her intention was not to take her participants from 0–100 in no time at all – and by that I mean from deep breathing straight into heavy back squats. She was simply trying to remove some of the stresses of their day, via diaphragmatic breathing, before starting their class with a thorough warm up, ensuring they got the most out of the session. If sleeping helps you to have better thoughts – improved cognitive function for the win – then diaphragmatic breathing helps you to collect your thoughts.

EVERYDAY MOVEMENT

If starting to increase the amount of movement in your life seems daunting, it can be comforting to think instead of what you are already doing. NEAT (see definition box) is the amount of energy we expend that is not exercise, eating or sleeping. All the other activities you do in your day – walking, moving around, cleaning, commuting, etc – all contribute to your daily NEAT. Why does it matter? Well, so much importance and emphasis is put on that one golden hour that you spend in the gym, that we act as if the other hours you spend just living don't count for anything. Well, they do! Everything matters: sleep, breathing, non-exercise movement. It's important to count all your daily activities as movement, even if those activities don't happen in the gym. Here are some ways we can fit a bit more NEAT into our daily lives:

HOUSE WORK: wash the dishes, do the hoovering, sweep up. Put your favourite music on, roll up your sleeves and get to it.

WALK TO YOUR DESTINATION: trade the tube for your feet. If your commute is too long to walk all the way, get off one stop early and walk the last bit.

MOBILE MEETING: try trading your meeting over lunch or coffee for a walking meeting – grab your phone, put your headphones in and take it outside.

GET UP: if you have a desk job, fitting mobility exercises into your day is key. Or just get up every hour and have a walk around.

SET A MOVEMENT ALARM: if you tend to forget to move for long periods of time (see point 4!), set an alarm to remind you to move regularly.

TAKE FLIGHT: five floors up? No problem. If you are physically able, use the stairs.

I know the exercises in the list above may seem trivial, especially when I've been holding back on the movement you've all been craving for. However, the everyday movement really matters and shouldn't be taken for granted; just like our mindset work, creating awareness around the stuff we already do that impacts our health will be a game changer.

OK, I think we're good – now we're ready to take on movement as you know it in the next chapter.

CHAPTER 4

MOVEMENT MATTERS

Wait . . . Stop it. We're here? Finally! Yes we are. Now let's go!

As I've discussed in chapter 3, we know that as we go about our day-to-day lives, we are constantly on the move; even when we are standing still, our muscles are working to keep us upright. When we take the stairs, we are moving primarily through our knees; when we pick up something heavy from the floor, we are moving primarily through our hips. Just by being active in our daily life, we already know what it is to 'move it'. We can pick up poor movement habits though, maybe slouching through our posture when standing or seated. When we don't move our bodies in the way we were designed to, we lose the ability to move efficiently in those positions, which can lead to aches, pains and injuries. My aim as a coach is to make sure you are moving your body as efficiently as you can; you will be more energised and feel better as a result.

FUNDAMENTAL MOVEMENT PATTERNS

Us trainers like to categorise movement in patterns; patterns help us to formulate specific exercises and programmes. Every waking moment, you are combining lots of different movement patterns to get about. If we can break it down and improve movement in each pattern, then it's fair to say we will be functioning better as a whole when those movements are combined together. We organise movement into the following patterns, depending on the action in the body: 'hip dominant', 'knee dominant', 'pull', 'push' and 'rotation'. Breaking general movement down in this way helps us to organise and prescribe exercises safely for the individual. To understand what these patterns look like, both in the gym and in the day-to-day activities you may be more familiar with, see the chart below.

MOVEMENT	IN THE GYM	IN REAL LIFE
Hip dominant	Deadlift	Picking something heavy up from the floor
Knee dominant	Lunge	Taking the stairs
Pull (horizontal)	Row	Opening a door
Pull (vertical)	Pull up	Climbing a tree
Push (horizontal)	Push up	Pushing anything in front of you

MOVEMENT	IN THE GYM	IN REAL LIFE
Push (vertical)	Overhead press	Placing something on a high shelf
Rotation	Windmills	Reaching behind you

Ideally, we should be able to demonstrate good movement in each pattern for our bodies to function well, but life gets in the way (sitting down all day, slouching, poor movement habits) and our posture and movements become a reflection of that. I don't set myself up with my feet and spine in a certain position as I sit down at my desk, as I would in a back squat; I just sit down without thinking – and then often stay there all day, whether I am in a healthy position or not. If I pick something small up off the ground, I might let out a grimace because bending feels a bit stiff, but other than that I may not think about it. If I pick something heavy up off the ground without thinking about it, I might regret it.

However, in a structured exercise setting, we can get specific about each movement pattern and choose the exercises that are most appropriate for a person's ability at that moment in time. It makes sense to pay attention to moving well in the gym, because it will come in handy in the day to day. When we throw dumbbells, kettlebells, barbells, maces and Indian clubs into the mix, we start to have some real fun with these movement patterns, as you will see when I introduce you to the mobility and strength exercises in the following chapters.

TAILORED TO YOU

Understanding the logic of a movement pattern means we can make it simpler or more complex for each individual, so that everyone is meeting their needs, no matter what their level or ability. It's particularly beneficial if someone is just starting out, coming back from an injury or has a physical disability, as we can always meet them where they are at.

So, in practising this movement, what exercise should you do? If you want to move well, you need to be aware of which exercises belong to each movement category. If you are only doing exercises that belong in two to three fundamental movement patterns, you are missing the good stuff from the other movement patterns to balance it all out! If you play sport, this matters even more, as you'll want to move really well in the dominant movement patterns of your sport. For example, if you are a boxer, you'll want to be able to rotate, push and have powerful hip dominant movement; as well as creating strength and balance through the movement patterns less used. We all need to give a nod to all of the movement patterns, as much as our physical ability allows. From this, we can understand that exercise isn't just exercise; we need to be smart in how we approach it.

A COMPLETE APPROACH

I ran two marathons in my early twenties. For the first, all I did to prepare for it was run. As I clocked up the miles in training, I saw a physio regularly to help treat the knee pain I was experiencing. During the race itself, I barked 'I'm never fucking doing this again' at my husband BJ around mile twenty – what a way to show gratitude for him darting around London to various milestones to support me! To get ready for that race, I mainly focused on cardiovascular fitness and recovery; I paid attention to cardiovascular fitness by running a lot. I recovered by making sure I was eating enough, getting enough sleep, taking ice baths after long runs, and getting massages when I could. But I let the other two – strength and mobility – go by the wayside. As I got closer to the race, a niggling knee pain got worse and I spent many sessions on a physio couch, with acupuncture needles in my legs and bum. Had I paid more attention to my mobility and strength this wouldn't have happened.

Fast forward a year, and the things I neglected were a priority – I was now focusing on my strength and mobility as well as cardiovascular fitness and recovery. I raced without knee pain, finished strong and was less sore the following day. I use this in the context of a race, but what I call 'the big four' are all equally important not just when moving it, but for everyday life. There are no shortcuts when we demand more of our bodies, and a little maintenance goes a long way if we want to move through each day feeling sweet.

THE BIG FOUR

The following are the four areas that I believe we need to pay attention to when it comes to movement:

MOBILITY – being able to safely control our joints through full range of motion.

STRENGTH – the ability to produce force against a resistance – from holding ourselves upright against gravity to lifting heavy weights or engaging in strenuous activity.

ENERGY SYSTEMS – our ability to utilise our cardiovascular system (the heart and blood vessels) for the demands of our energy output – walking, climbing and moving around in general.

RECOVERY – intentional practices to allow our bodies to recuperate from physical and mental exertion.

Over the next four chapters I will cover each one of these in turn, to help you incorporate more movement into your life in a healthy way.

And because I love you a lot, recovery plays a particularly important part, encompassing sleep and breathing, which we have already covered – we are coming full circle!

CHAPTER 5

MOBILITY

Can you get up and down from the floor without using your hands? Try it. It's kind of fun but it shows what is required to be mobile, to have strength and flexibility at the same time. This should be simple. I don't say this to make you feel inadequate, but a fully mobile body would be able to do this easily. I'm willing to bet that most people who don't actively do mobility work will find the task hard, so you and I are in this together – I grunted, too!

If we look at the body as a whole, we have joints whose primary role is to be mobile – the thoracic spine, hip and ankle; and we have joints whose primary role is to be stable – the cervical spine, lumbar spine and knee.

When joints that are supposed to be mobile lose their mobility, we run into issues. Our bodies are incredible compensators; if one area isn't doing its job, the same demands will be made of an unsuspecting neighbour – but those demands will be made in addition to them doing their actual job, and so extra strain is put on the body.

Let's apply this. Take a look at the top you're wearing; we're going to use it as an example of what can happen when we're not mobile.

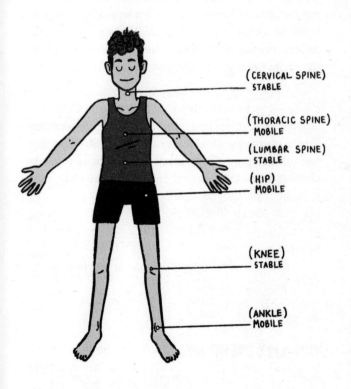

(CERVICAL SPINE)
STABLE

(THORACIC SPINE)
MOBILE

(LUMBAR SPINE)
STABLE

(HIP)
MOBILE

(KNEE)
STABLE

(ANKLE)
MOBILE

71

Flatten your top out, as if you have spilt crumbs down yourself (or is that just me?), then grab a small part of it and turn it clockwise. What happens to the rest of the fabric? It's turned and pulled with it, right? You may even feel the collar of your top now pulling on the back of your neck. This is similar to the experience your body goes through.

When one area of the body is not mobile enough, other areas take the brunt, so quite often the site where you are feeling pain is not necessarily the direct source of it. In the example of your top, that pull you feel on the back of your neck is actually coming from the front of your body. This can lead to aches, pains and potential injuries, but it can also just mean that we don't feel as good moving around as we potentially could. If we are limited in our range of movement, we can't fully access our strength (and you're about to read why I practically have a corner in my house where I pray to the strength gods. We absolutely want full access to our strength! It's the shit!).

MOBILITY EXERCISES

Here are some of my favourite mobility exercises. They should take an average of five minutes. Taking that amount of time to work through these daily will allow you a dedicated moment to check in with your body. While you're doing this, be sure to include some diaphragmatic breathing (see page 55) – see, it's all coming together nicely, isn't it?

I recommend you read these through twice before starting. Your set up is your starting position; how you set yourself up before you begin is important as we want to start every movement from a good position and with intention.

EXERCISE I: Adductor rockback with rotation

SET UP: Starting on all fours, take your right leg out to the side, keeping your right foot in line with your left knee.

1. Slowly push your hips back towards your heel – you will feel a stretch through your right inner thigh and left groin. Rock back and forth slowly.

---

2. After three repetitions, place your right hand by your right ear, then reach your right elbow towards your left elbow, then away from your left elbow towards the ceiling, so that you are rotating through your spine.

REPEAT this for 3–4 repetitions, then do the same on the other side.

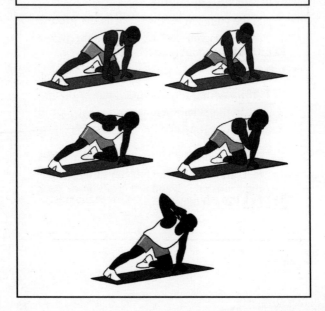

EXERCISE 2: The world's greatest stretch

SET UP: Stand with your feet underneath your hips. With a soft bend in the knees, place your hands on the floor and slowly walk your hands out into a top plank.

1. Place your left foot on the outside of the left hand, doing your best to ensure the whole of the left foot is on the ground.

2. Place your left elbow towards the ground as best as you can, then rotate the whole of the left arm towards the ceiling.

3. Place the left hand back on the outside of the left foot, then take the foot back to meet the right so that you are back in a top plank position.

4. Slowly walk the hands back towards the feet, and curl back up to standing.

REPEAT the whole routine on the right side.

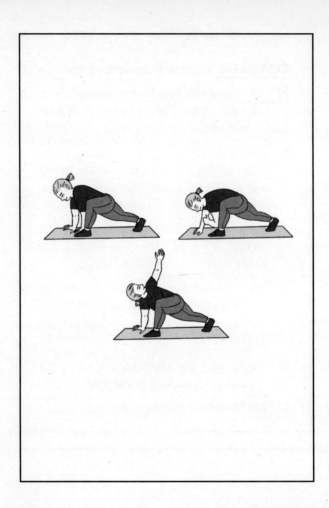

EXERCISE 3: Shinbox switch into extension

SET UP: Sit on the ground with your legs bent and feet flat on the floor, and hands behind you for support.

1. Let both knees fall over to the right, ensuring they are both at a 90-degree angle. Keeping your hands on the ground, lower both knees over to the left. Move back and forth from right to left. If it feels comfortable for you to do so, you can take your hands off the ground so that they are no longer providing support.

2. If step 1 feels good, after you drop the knees to the right, lift your hips off the ground so you are now in a tall kneeling position; then sit the hips back down, rotate the knees over to the left and lift your hips off the ground so you are in a tall kneeling position.

3. If step 2 feels good, bring the knees back over to the right, lift the hips up to a tall kneeling position, then step the left foot forward past the right knee so you are in a kneeling lunge. Then take the left foot back to the tall kneeling position, and sit the hips back down. Repeat on the left side to extend the hips and step the right foot forward into a kneeling lunge.

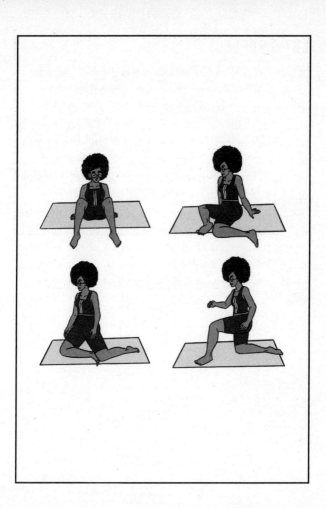

LET'S REFLECT

What did you notice when you did these exercises? Is one side easier than the other? It's all just information, you don't need to worry that one side feels less mobile than the other. You just know your body a little better now, and you can breathe deeper into these mobility exercises now that you know. Oh, and that last exercise is preparation for you getting up off the floor without using your hands. You're welcome! These are all fairly big moves as you get to mobilise lots of different joints at the same time, but you can also break mobility down into a joint by joint approach, by moving one joint at a time: your neck, your left hip, your right hip, etc.

CHAPTER 6

STRENGTH

One sec, I'm just going to nip to that corner of my house where I pray to the strength gods. Done. Thanks for being patient. OK, how do I put this – quite simply, strength is everything. Ev-er-y-thing. And if there is a fear that strength training will turn you into Arnold Schwarzenegger, let me stop you there. Strong doesn't necessarily mean you will look muscly, and looking muscly doesn't necessarily mean you are strong. I used to compete in local strength and power competitions in my early thirties. You would throw around heavy, odd-shaped objects and get to do random stuff like pull cars and vans (apparently there's a video of me out there). In these exercises we did fun stuff you don't get to do in a regular gym.

A few friends of mine were competing with me, and we sat together sizing up the competition. 'She looks good,' I thought looking at one girl, 'got her covered.' looking at another. Well, shame on me for judging my competition based on their looks because the slight-framed girl who didn't *look* like she had any muscle ended up wiping the floor with all of us. She was as strong as hell and gave me the whooping I deserved for thinking I didn't need to worry about her. Karma, eh? I've never made that mistake again.

I run strength workshops exclusively for women with my friend Lisa Price. Strength training built my confidence in a way I could never have anticipated, but access to it can be limited for those who find gyms intimidating spaces. We wanted to give access to women so they too could benefit from the feeling that being strong brings.

At the start of the workshop we always ask the room, 'Who is worried about getting too muscly?' A few sheepish hands always rise up; we take note and look forward to them meeting their own strength for the first time by the end of the day. After a full warm up by Lisa, whose way of teaching is like poetry, we go through the three main lifts: the squat, the deadlift and the press. When executed well, there is a lot to think about. Part of the beauty of strength training is building a movement relationship with your body; I'd go as far as saying it's a journey. By the end, they understand any movement limitations they may have, have a sense of their strength capacity and a new-found respect for what their bodies can do!

For me as a coach, seeing a client realise their own strength is incredible, and it never gets old. The shock of their achievement is infectious: 'Wait, I just lifted that? My body just did that?' Yes, it did! And look, you did it, and your biceps didn't just bust out of your sleeves and attack you! Strength is that one thing that people can't take away from you. You own it. And that's priceless.

However, we can also lose strength. Either through:

1. **NON-USE:** 'Use it, or lose it'. Our bodies are efficient with where they direct energy – you're not using it? OK, let's shut that down.

2. <u>AGE</u>: We start to lose muscle mass in our early thirties.

Losing our strength matters because so many aspects of our health benefit from it – bone density, metabolic rate, physical function, cardiovascular health, cognitive function, mental health, pain reduction, injury prevention and the ageing process.

Why do I personally love strength training so much? To make the most out of it, you have to go inward (here she goes again). Breathe, think about the set up, and ask yourself: 'What does my body need to do in order to perform this movement safely?' And the barbell never lies. If the weight doesn't move, you're not ready. Mercury isn't in retrograde, you're just not ready. You could be having an off day (after a bad night's sleep, or during your menstrual cycle, etc.) or it could be that you have expected too much of your body before it is ready.

STRENGTH EXERCISES

So where and how do I make these gains? I promise you it doesn't involve you packed into a weight room with an abundance of biceps and pecs staring at you. Managing your own bodyweight first without any external loading is where we start. Think squats, lunges, push ups. Common but not easy. I'll say that again for the people at the back. Common but not easy! Just because you're not lifting any weight yet, doesn't mean you can chill. No equipment is required just yet, so you don't even need to set foot outside the door. (I know, I'm the gift that keeps on giving with this strength vibe.)

For each movement there are levels. We start with the safest first – this may mean starting from the floor on all fours or in a position where we don't have to think about too many things at once – and then slowly build to more complex, dynamic movement that requires good movement control so that we are still safe if we are moving fast or doing a movement that does several things at once. We can liken it to how a baby first learns to move: crawling, standing with support, walking and finally running – each developmental process is more complex than the previous version of the same movement pattern. The more conscientious you are about building good movement patterns at the start, the better off you will be!

Here are three movements that you can get going with straight away, along with progressions of the movements in case you're getting antsy and just want to throw some weight around already. Before you start, warm up with the mobility drills from chapter 5, and complete 3–4 repetitions on each side.

EXERCISE I: Active quadruped

SET UP: You will need a foam roller, water bottle or anything cylindrical. Position yourself on all fours, then place the roller horizontally across your lower back.

1. Lift your knees one inch off the ground and focus on keeping the roller on your back.

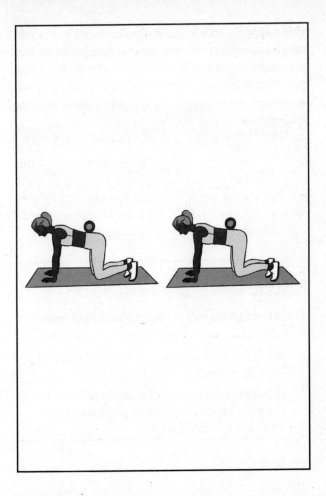

The following are some progressions of the active quadruped. They do not have to be performed in this order – they are just examples of how you could progress this movement.

MOVEMENT	PROGRESSION 1	PROGRESSION 2	PROGRESSION 3	PROGRESSION 4
Active quadruped	Foam roller bear crawl	Lateral foam roller bear crawl	Weighted (in hands) foam roller bear crawl	Resisted (plate attached from behind) bear crawl

PROGRESSION 1: FOAM ROLLER BEAR CRAWL

SET UP: Start off in the 'active quadruped position' (see page 86).

1. Take a small step forward with your left hand and right foot at the same time; then continue a step forward with your right hand and your left foot at the same time. Take care to keep the foam roller on your back throughout.

2. You can continue this forward movement with small continuous steps forward, or you can take a few steps forward, followed by a few steps backwards.

Do this for 30–60 seconds or for as long as you can keep the foam roller on your back without it falling off.

PROGRESSION 2: LATERAL FOAM ROLLER BEAR CRAWL

SET UP: Start off in the 'active quadruped position' (see page 86).

1. Take a small step sideways to the left with your left hand and right foot at the same time; then continue a step to the left with your right hand and your left foot at the same time. Take care to keep the foam roller on your back throughout.

2. Continue this lateral movement for 2–3 more steps to the left, then repeat moving to the right.

Do this for 30–60 seconds in each direction or for as long as you can keep the foam roller on your back without it falling off.

PROGRESSION 3: WEIGHTED FOAM ROLLER BEAR CRAWL

SET UP: Holding a 1–3kg dumbbell in each hand, start off in the 'active quadruped position' (see page 86), ensuring your wrists are straight.

1. Take a small step forward with your left hand and right foot at the same time; then continue a step forward with your right hand and your left foot at the same time. Take care to keep the foam roller on your back throughout.

2. You can continue this forward movement with small continuous steps forward, or you can take a few steps forward, followed by a few steps backwards.

Do this for 30–60 seconds or for as long as you can keep the foam roller on your back without it falling off.

PROGRESSION 4: RESISTED BEAR CRAWL

SET UP: Start off in the 'active quadruped position' (see page 86) with a small weight plate attached to you via a weight belt, or a thick resistance band around your waist (do not use the foam roller in this version).

1. Take a small step forward with your left hand and right foot at the same time; then continue a step forward with your right hand and your left foot at the same time. Continue this forward movement with small steps forward.

Do this for 30–60 seconds.

EXERCISE 2: Split squat

SET UP: Have a chair, table or broom as support. Place your left hand on your support. Start from standing with your right leg a few feet in front of your left.

1. Ensuring the whole of your right foot is in contact with the ground, slowly sink your left knee towards the ground, keeping your chest nice and upright.

2. Slowly return to standing. It's OK for there to be a slight forward lean in your upper body, but if you were doing this facing the mirror you should still be able to see the pocket of your t-shirt (imagine one

---

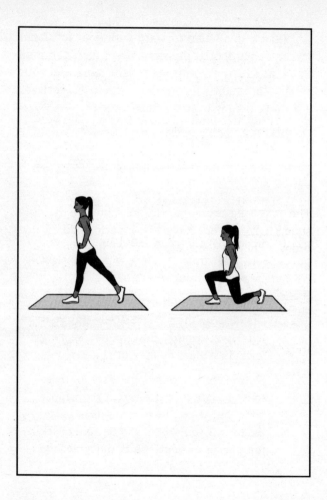

if there is no pocket). If it is comfortable for you to do it without holding onto anything, do so.

REPEAT this for 8–10 repetitions on the right side, then do the same on the left.

The following are some progressions of the split squat. They do not have to be performed in this order – they are just examples of how you could progress this movement.

MOVEMENT	PROGRESSION 1	PROGRESSION 2	PROGRESSION 3	PROGRESSION 4
Split squat	Front foot elevated (FFE) split squat	Reverse lunge	Goblet reverse lunge	Forward lunge

PROGRESSION 1: FRONT FOOT ELEVATED SPLIT SQUAT

SET UP: Have a thick book, yoga block or weight plate on the ground in front of you. Start from standing with your right foot on the book/block/plate a few feet in front of your left foot, which will be on the ground.

1. Ensuring the whole of your right foot is in contact with the base you are standing on, slowly sink your left knee towards the ground, keeping your chest upright.

2. Return to standing.

REPEAT this for 8–10 repetitions on the right side, then do the same on the left.

PROGRESSION 2: REVERSE LUNGE

SET UP: Stand tall with your feet hip-width apart.

1. Take a large step back with your left leg, letting the left knee lower down towards the floor – both knees should be bent to roughly 90 degrees with your torso remaining upright.

2. Stand back up by placing your bodyweight through your right foot and stepping forward with the left so that both feet end up hip-width apart again.

REPEAT this for 6–8 repetitions on the right side, then do the same on the left.

PROGRESSION 3: GOBLET REVERSE LUNGE

SET UP: Hold a dumbbell vertically with your hands cupping the upper base, or a kettlebell upside down (as if you were cupping a wine glass with both your hands). Stand tall with your feet hip-width apart.

1. Take a large step back with your left leg, letting the left knee lower down towards the floor – both knees should be bent to roughly 90 degrees with your torso remaining upright.

2. Stand back up by placing your bodyweight through your right foot and stepping forward with the left so that both feet end up hip-width apart again.

REPEAT this for 6–8 repetitions on the right side, then do the same on the left.

PROGRESSION 4 – FORWARD LUNGE

SET UP: Stand tall with your feet hip-width apart.

1. Take a large step forward with your left leg, letting your right knee lower down towards the floor – both knees should be bent to roughly 90 degrees with your torso remaining upright.

2. Stand back up by pushing your weight through the heel of your left foot as you return to the start position. Imagine that there are train tracks in front of you, and each time you step forward you are keeping both feet in line with the train tracks – this will ensure you maintain the correct stance width as you move in and out of the lunge.

REPEAT this for 6–8 repetitions on the left side, then do the same on the right.

EXERCISE 3: Squat to box

SET UP: Stand in front of a chair or bench with your feet slightly wider than hip-width apart and slightly turned out to create a little

---

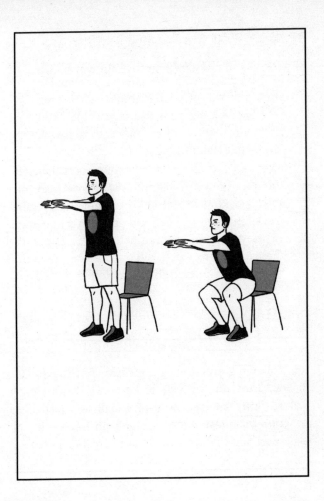

extra space in your hips. Ensure both feet are in full contact with the ground by thinking about the ball of your foot (an inch behind your big toe), the outer ball of your foot (half an inch behind your baby toe) and your heel, then think about trying to spread the ground with your feet (keeping those three points of contact) – you will feel how active your legs and feet feel when you do this.

1. Lower your hips slowly towards the chair making contact with it without sitting down

2. Stand back up, keeping those three points of contact with the ground throughout.

REPEAT this for 8–10 repetitions.

The following are some progressions of the squat to box. They do not have to be performed in this order – they are just examples of how you could progress this movement.

MOVEMENT	PROGRESSION 1	PROGRESSION 2	PROGRESSION 3	PROGRESSION 4
Squat to box	Bodyweight squat	Goblet squat	Front squat	Back squat

PROGRESSION 1: BODYWEIGHT SQUAT

SET UP: Stand as you did in the squat to box, only you will not need the chair this time.

1. Imagining the chair behind you, slowly lower down into a squat.

2. Stand back up, keeping those three points of contact with the ground throughout.

REPEAT this for 8-10 repetitions.

NOTE: If you find that your torso falls forward, you can try doing the squat facing a wall, or place your hands by your ears – both may help you to keep your torso a little more upright.

PROGRESSION 2: GOBLET SQUAT

SET UP: Hold a dumbbell vertically with your hands cupping the upper base, or a kettlebell upside down (as if you were cupping a wine glass with both your hands). Stand as you did in the squat to box, only you will not need the chair this time.

1. Letting your knees and hips flex at the same time, slowly lower your hips back and down into a squat.

2. Stand back up, keeping those three points of contact with the ground throughout.

REPEAT this for 8-10 repetitions.

NOTE: Having the kettlebell in front of you will help keep your torso more upright if you feel it falls forward in the bodyweight squat.

PROGRESSION 3: FRONT SQUAT

SET UP: Place a barbell in a squat rack set lower than your shoulder height. Approach the bar, take a quarter squat, then put your arms straight out in front of you so the bar is resting on your shoulders. With your right hand, grip the bar on the inside of your left shoulder, then with your left hand, grip the bar on the inside of your right shoulder.

Stand the bar up, keeping your elbows up and maintaining the firm grip with your hands. Take a step back out of the squat rack, and take your feet out slightly wider than hip-width apart, with your toes slightly turned out to give you a little more space in your hips.

1. Letting your knees and hips flex at the same time, slowly lower your hips down into a squat, focusing on keeping the elbows raised the whole time.

2. Stand back up, keeping those three points of contact with the ground throughout.

REPEAT this for 8-10 repetitions.

NOTE: The crossarm position given above is great for beginners who may not have the shoulder mobility to hold the traditional front rack position of hands placed on the outside of the same-side shoulder.

PROGRESSION 4: BACK SQUAT

SET UP: Place a barbell in a squat rack set lower than your shoulder height. Approach the bar, take a quarter squat, and step under the bar, placing your hands in an overhand grip outside of your shoulders; squeeze your shoulder blades together to create a shelf on the back of your shoulders to rest the bar on. Pulling down firmly on the bar to secure it to the shelf created by your shoulders, and ensuring your feet are under your hips, stand the bar up and step out of the rack. Take your feet out slightly wider than shoulder-width apart, with your toes slightly turned out to give you a little more space in your hips.

1. Letting your knees and hips flex at the same time, slowly lower your hips down into a squat.

2. Stand back up, keeping those three points of contact with the ground throughout.

REPEAT this for 8-10 repetitions.

TIPS AND TRICKS

Here are some tips and tricks to help you with your first foray into strength exercises.

FIND YOUR FEET

Standing properly on your feet is important in strength training. If we think of our feet as our foundation, we want to make sure that foundation is securely planted so we can move well or add load. Try this little experiment. Stand and place your weight towards the front of your feet; now try it again with your weight placed towards the back of your feet. Do you feel stable in either of these positions? Unless you have your weight centred over your feet, you are off balance. When we are training, what happens at our feet can be a lot more subtle, but it is still not optimal. So now do the squat to box again, this time focusing on those three points of contact. The ball of your foot (an inch behind your big toe), the outer ball of your foot (half an inch behind your baby toe) and your heel should all be in contact with the ground. Think about trying to spread the ground with your feet (keeping those three points of contact) – you will feel how active your legs and feet feel when you do this. As you sit down towards the chair, are you maintaining that tension in your feet, or has your focus now drifted to your bum finding the chair? So many things to think about, right? Don't worry, with practice this all gets easier and will become second nature. But in the beginning as you build these good movement habits, you really have to think about it; you're really drilling in that mind–muscle connection.

POWER FROM YOUR CORE

Gymnasts spend a large portion of their training working the hollow body position – using their core as the stable centre point with both arms and legs extended. This is the foundation for all gymnastic movements, whether in a handstand, on the rings, or tumbling across the floor. It's fairly common these days in gyms, but executed questionably because it's difficult to do well. The basics are not basic, but they are skipped in favour of something more complex because that's the sexy stuff (cries a little inside). When you did the active quadruped, the only thing that kept that foam roller from falling off your back will have been your 'core' muscles working. Now the beauty of using the foam roller is that it does the thinking for you. What if I had asked you to do that same exercise without the foam roller. You would have breezed it, right? On all fours, knees hovering above the ground. 'This is easy, Joslyn, I am awesome!' Except that roller made you check yourself, in the nicest possible way. You were out there shaking and sweating with the roller outing you as soon as you lost control. To the naked eye, it doesn't look like much. But inside, there were big why-am-I-shaking-so-much tears. It's OK. But don't miss this part. Foundations are everything.

TEMPO IS YOUR FRIEND

'The slower you go, the more control you have.' If you have ever been a client of mine, you will have eye-rolled at me constantly repeating those words.

Slowing movement down forces your body to figure out where it needs to be in time and space. For the flexible among you, you may be able to fling yourself into a bodyweight squat without so much as a care and be like, 'And what? This is easy!' Let's just strip that back, shall we? If the foam roller reveals the truth of your core control – or the lack thereof – slowing stuff down will force you to face the bits that you skipped because you were flexible enough to get there. See, here's the problem: let's say you can dive bomb into a bodyweight squat and there you are, your butt close to the floor, and me all like, wow, what a great squat – let me load her up, it was so easy for her to get there. Except, because you got there so quickly, your body may not know how to do it safely. It's kind of OK unloaded in a bodyweight squat, maybe even with a light load. But when we add more weight, we start to add more pressure to your joints. Combine this with you not paying attention to your feet and your core, and we have ourselves a problem. Best case, you get stuck in the bottom of a barbell back squat and you have some pals to help you outta there. Worst case, you get stuck in the bottom of a barbell back squat and you have some pals to help you outta there, except you've herniated a disc in your spine and you're out of that type of training for a long ass time. That or some other injury that will put a wee pause on your speedy bodyweight squat prowess. So it's important to be able to demonstrate that you can move under control, even if you're fast and fly. You're great, but I want you to stay great. So first we go slow.

As you do more in the way of training, you can get really specific with tempo as a way of adding variety to an exercise, by adjusting the speed at which you do a movement.

CHAPTER 7

ENERGY SYSTEMS

What do you envision when you think of cardio – running, cycling, swimming, rowing? Yes, it is all of those things, but so much more. Its heyday in popular culture from the seventies to the nineties made sweatbands the accessory of choice and aerobics classes were the place to be seen. Fast forward to now and the idea of aerobics is largely laughed at as we favour high intensity interval training (HIIT) and strength (which we love, obviously, but the other stuff is still important). Cardiovascular fitness is the use of different energy systems. Both aerobics and HIIT utilise the cardiovascular system but in different ways and intensities. If you use a heart rate monitor (which tracks the pace of your heart beats per minute), you can also count lifting weights as cardio if you're working in the right heart rate zones.

There are three main energy systems that make up the cardiovascular system – aerobic, anaerobic (lactic acid) and anaerobic (creatine phosphate). Different types of movement require different energy demands and so your body draws on three different energy systems to select the most appropriate source. An activity such as sprinting, which requires a high energy demand of maximum force and power, will utilise energy generated from a different system to a long walk or jog, which requires a much lower level of intensity but for a much longer period.

AEROBIC – This is the lowest amount of energy output required from our bodies and so can be done for an extended period of time. Doing an activity for 3 minutes or more will utilise our aerobic system. This includes most activities we do daily – think back to non-exercise activity thermogenesis (NEAT) on page 58.

ANAEROBIC – LACTIC ACID SYSTEM – A medium to high amount of energy output required; doing an activity for 10 seconds to 3 minutes will utilise our lactic acid system. The energy output required is greater than the aerobic system (think 400m sprints), but the time is limited from 10 seconds to 3 minutes due to the increase in energy required.

ANAEROBIC – CREATINE PHOSPHATE (CP) – A maximum amount of energy output required, limiting the activity to just 1–10 seconds. Think an all-out sprint – our body can only sustain this for a very short amount of time and will utilise our lactic acid system for the energy. The shorter and more intense the output, the longer the time required for recovery.

These three systems don't work exclusively, but one dominates at different times. I want to focus on aerobic capacity: cardiac output specifically. This is long, slow training, so great to start with if you are new (but equally important for everyone) and it's the secret behind everything. See, everybody is going hard and fast, not realising that time spent in the slow intensity lane at least once a week will improve the capacity of all three systems. Yep, going slow helps you to go faster at a higher intensity for longer and recover quicker. I know!

OK, so let me just get this out of my system real quick. Do not judge the effectiveness of a workout by how much you sweat. Write that down and remember it. It's the biggest misconception that exists in the world of fitness. Any fool can make you sweat; it doesn't display the skill of the coach and doesn't determine the efficiency of your workout. And I get it – when you feel that burn and there are droplets of sweat coming out of your pores, something has to be happening, right? Yes, something is happening. You are sweating and feeling hot. If we consider some of the most elite athletes in the world and look at their training across the week, month or year, those sweat opportunities exist less than you would think, and you can bet they get all the sleep, do all the mobility and spend time getting strong in the gym. Except somehow we mistakenly associate fitness with sweating.

So how do we develop our cardiac output if it doesn't mean sweating up a storm and collapsing in a heap? Spending time in a heart rate zone loosely between 120–150 beats per minute will increase your cardiac output. The fitter you are, the more you should veer towards the lower end of 120–130 bpm (because your heart will already be efficient at pumping blood, so can do it at a slower pace); and the less conditioned you are, you will find yourself working near the higher end of 140–150 bpm (because it will take a while for movement to not be as demanding on your cardiovascular system, so your heart will be working harder to pump blood). In general, the fitter you are, the more efficient your heart is at pumping blood around your body, so the slower it beats.

Training in this heart rate zone of 120–150 bpm for at least 30 minutes 1–3 times per week will increase your cardiac output. You can build all the way up to 90 minutes if you are keen – your health will thank you for it. The more you train in this zone, the more efficient your heart becomes at pumping blood around your body. This is useful because it helps you recover more quickly, it helps you go harder for longer, and it increases your overall work capacity. Winning! And you know I am all about building foundations that build the things!

So where do we start on this cardio journey? Are you lacing up your shoes ready for a little jaunt outside? Brilliant, I love your enthusiasm, but hold up. Working your aerobic system with a view to building cardiac output requires you to do any type of movement – yes, anything – as long as it is continuous and keeps you in that heart rate zone: dancing, mobilising, uphill walking, even weight training. And if you haven't got a heart rate monitor, it's cool, I got you – you can utilise what's known as your rate of perceived exertion. This is a measure of the level of intensity you are working at and is a good alternative to heart rate training.

RATE OF PERCEIVED EXERTION (RPE)

Rate of perceived exertion is your interpretation, in the moment, of how intense something feels. Let's break it down into levels from your sofa to the gym:

LEVEL 1: I'm watching Netflix and expending zero energy.

LEVEL 2: I'm chill, moving about my day, no stress.

LEVEL 3: I'm cool but breathing a little harder cos I'm moving about with a little extra juice.

LEVEL 4: I'm sweating a little, but I can still talk easily.

LEVEL 5: A little less chill, am sweating more but can still talk easily.

LEVEL 6: Less chat from me now and a little more breathless.

LEVEL 7: One-word answers, OK! Pass me a towel, my sweat is in full flow.

LEVEL 8: Starting to hurt, no chat, how long?

LEVEL 9: OK, all the hurt, I cannot sustain this!

LEVEL 10: I'm done, stop! Did I just die?

If we look at the different types of cardio and categorised them into rate of perceived exertion, we could say:

— Aerobic would sit between level 1–4; working our cardiac output would sit between 3–4.

- Anaerobic lactic acid would sit between level 5–7.

- Anaerobic creatine phosphate (CP) would be over level 8.

So whatever type of movement you choose to do to build cardiac output, ensure that it is continuous for at least 30 minutes and that it has the feels of level 3, 'I'm cool but breathing a little harder cos I'm moving about with a little extra juice', and level 4, 'I'm sweating a little, but I can still talk easily'.

I want to put a final note in here about walking. If you still have it in your mind that things like jogging are 'real' cardio but don't feel ready to do that, walk. Walking is one of the most underrated yet effective forms of movement there is. Not only is it good for blood flow and therefore good for your heart, it is also fantastic for clearing your mind too. When we walk, we are generally not on our phones or distracted by other things. We can bundle it up with the wise advice of 'just breathe' and 'sleep on it' – 'take a walk to clear your mind' does exactly what it says on the tin. If I am stressed and have some time, I will walk. In fact, when I am stressed and even if I don't have time, I will walk: it *always* helps. So, start with walking if you wish. If you want to work your cardiac output, walk briskly – your mind and heart will both thank you.

If you want to follow a specific plan for increasing cardiovascular fitness, turn to my workouts in chapter 9 for some simple programmes to get you started.

CHAPTER 8

RECOVERY

Recovery is the flag I fly the most, even as someone who is obsessed with movement. Exercise is good for you but it's also a stress: a good stress if life isn't throwing too many other stresses at you; but a bad stress if you are already stressed out in other areas of your life. This is really common in the person who is stressed at home and at work and so trains to de-stress. There may be some short-term relief, but in the long term this will lead to potential illness or injury if the body is unable to recover. Let's revisit the autonomic nervous system again to see why.

As I discussed in chapter 3, we have the sympathetic system and the parasympathetic system. The sympathetic system we refer to as 'fight or flight' because it puts us into a state of readiness for action: our heart rate and blood pressure increase; we sweat more (think sweaty palms); blood is redirected towards the muscles (so we can move fast); the bladder relaxes (think nervous wee); and digestion is inhibited. There is a lot going on! Again, this really served us when we were being chased by lions before we then (hopefully) rested. But modern-day stress triggers the same hormonal response (work, exams, traffic, relationships, the internet) and we are in this sympathetic state of readiness over a much longer period of time.

The parasympathetic system we refer to as 'rest and digest' because it puts us into a state of recovery and restoration: the heart rate slows to conserve energy; tissues are repaired; and digestion increases. It's important we know how to stimulate the parasympathetic nervous system not only to reduce the impact of every day stressors, but also to allow us to enable adequate recovery and adaptation from exercise. The benefits of working out will not be realised if we are unable to sufficiently recover.

So where do we start? Well, lucky you, you already know one of the real important parts of that. Sing it . . . SLEEP! Could there be a more perfect state in which the parasympathetic system could do its job? While those little peepers are closed, your body does the real work. Change doesn't take place while you train, it takes place while you are resting: that relaxed state allows the parasympathetic nervous system to do its job. So if you are skipping on sleep, that workout you did isn't going to reach its full potential. It would be like mixing the most delicious ingredients together for a meal and forgetting to put it in the oven to see it come to fruition. The rest allows the work to really come into play. Here are some other ways to recover:

BREATHE: we've got this covered, right? It keeps us alive and stimulates the parasympathetic nervous system (see page 55). When you are stressed, it's a good idea to pay attention to your breathing; it may not change the outcome of what it is you are stressed about, but it may adjust your body's physiological response to it.

STAY HYDRATED: our bodies are made of up to 60% water. It is essential to every system and function in the body: it lubricates our joints; regulates body temperature; flushes out waste; forms saliva; is a building block of new cells; and is what every cell relies on for survival. Being dehydrated impacts all of the above, affecting our ability to think, perform and function. And no I don't care if you don't like the taste or it makes you pee more. Drink it. You need it. We can get fancy with measuring out exactly how much you need, but let's start with 6–8 glasses a day.

EAT GOOD WHOLE FOODS: such as vegetables, meat, fish, nuts and seeds. Food is where we get our energy from to move. The more nutrient-dense it is, the better you will function. (That's as far as we are going on nutrition, it's a whole book in itself!)

TAKE AN EPSOM SALT BATH: Epsom salts are made up of magnesium sulphate, which helps your muscles to relax. Use 300–400g in a bath and soak for 10–20 minutes. (it's like a massage in the bath, I kid you not)

HAVE A SAUNA: sauna bathing aids your recovery by increasing your circulation and delivering oxygen and nutrients to your cells. A good place to start is 15–20 minutes, 1–3 times per week.

COLD THERAPY: how do I put this ... have an ice bath. Yes – you, an ice bath. I promise you even a 1–3-minute cold shower will help you sleep like a baby. For a deep dive into the benefits, check out Wim Hof on cold therapy: he suggests it can improve sleep quality, sharpness of the mind and immune function.

The more you train, the more attention you need to pay to recovery. Seven years ago I learned of the 'recovery credit/debit system' UFC veteran Bobby Maximus uses, it's a smart system to make sure you never go a training week under-recovered. For every recovery activity you do, you credit yourself with recovery points, for example: 7-9 hours sleep = 5 points; hydration = 2 points; nutritious food = 3 points; Epsom salt bath = 2 points; meditation = 2 points; cold therapy = 2 points; massage = 3 points, etc. The more recovery you schedule into your week, the more points you have to play with. Then you have your debits: yep, your training. Intense sessions like a heavy lifting session, or 400m sprints, might cost you 10 points, whereas a light 20-minute walk or jog may only cost you 3 points. Either way, you should have enough recovery points stored up so that you can train without being in a recovery deficit.

I use this in my own training: the harder I train or the more stressful life is, the more attention I need to pay to recovery. It is OK to push yourself physically and therefore mentally, but that will come at a high price if you do so without paying attention to recovery.

I know many of you reading this are starting out on your fitness journey, but I'm going to assume that this is the first day of many and it would be useful for you to recognise the signs of doing too much in your training. Be mindful of the following: tiredness, low mood, lack of motivation, no improvements in strength or fitness, insomnia and getting ill often. These can all be signs that your body is not recovered enough to train. Develop your own credit/debit system and tally your own training and recovery; it's a useful tool and will support you on your training journey.

CHAPTER 9

THE WORKOUTS

I hope that by now you have a deeper appreciation of movement and why it matters. Below, you will find a simple bodyweight strength programme as well as a simple programme to build your cardiovascular fitness. Remember the 'mobility' aspect of the big four? This is part of your warm up in the strength programme. And don't forget to focus on recovery once you have done the movement programmes (see chapter 8).

I would recommend that you do the bodyweight strength programme once or twice a week, the cardiovascular fitness programme once or twice a week, and recover daily! There are beginner and intermediate versions of each programme, as well as workouts that add weights as you start to build your strength. Each programme should take between 15 and 20 minutes. Instructions for any exercises referred to in the programmes that have not already been covered in the previous chapters can be found at the end of this chapter.

BODYWEIGHT STRENGTH – BEGINNER

We will begin with bodyweight: no external load, just you mastering your bodyweight. It's important that we do this before adding any load. If we cannot do a movement well with just our bodyweight, then we have no business adding load.

WARM UP	MAIN WORKOUT	COOL DOWN
— Walk out (see page 145): 5 repetitions — World's greatest stretch (see page 75): 3 repetitions each side — Foam roller quadruped shoulder taps (see page 146): 10 repetitions each side	— Kneeling hip hinge (see page 136): 2–3 sets of 8–10 repetitions — Split squat (see page 91): 2–3 sets of 8–10 repetitions — Kneeling plank row (see page 136): 2–3 sets of 4 repetitions each side — Eccentric push up (see page 137): 2-3 sets of 1-2 repetitions	— World's greatest stretch: 3 repetitions each side — Scorpions with pec stretch (see page 138): 3 repetitions each side

To begin with, do your warm up, then run through all of the exercises in the main workout, doing the number of sets and repetitions listed. Rest as needed, then repeat one more time for a total of two sets. Once that feels comfortable, you can add a third set. As that starts to feel good you could try two of the exercises back to back as a 'superset'. You have lots of different ways you can play around with the same workout, whilst easily being able to measure your progress.

BODYWEIGHT STRENGTH – INTERMEDIATE

Once you feel competent with three sets of the main set of the beginner workout, you can move on to the intermediate bodyweight workout. We are still keeping the same fundamental movement patterns, but the movements themselves are a little more complex. There is no rush here, the more time you spend feeling good in these movements, the better. This is your journey, enjoy it. Strength takes time to build, there are no shortcuts.

WARM UP	MAIN WORKOUT	COOL DOWN
— Walk out (see page 145): 5 repetitions	— Tempo glute bridge (see page 139): 3–4 sets of 8–10 repetitions	— World's greatest stretch: 3 repetitons each side

WARM UP	MAIN WORKOUT	COOL DOWN
— World's greatest stretch (see page 75): 3 repetitions each side — Foam roller quadruped shoulder taps (see page 146): 10 repetitions each side	— Bulgarian split squat (see page 139): 3-4 sets of 5-6 repetitions on each leg — High plank row (see page 140): 3-4 sets of 4-5 repetitions on each side — Eccentric push up (see page 137): 2-3 sets of 2-3 repetitions	— Scorpions with pec stretch (see page 138): 3 repetitions each side

As we did with the beginner bodyweight workout, you can start with two sets of the main set. Once that feels comfortable, you can add a third and even a fourth set. As that starts to feel good, you could try two of the exercises back to back as a 'superset'. Or you could play around with the speed at which you execute the movement: for example, lower down in an eccentric push up for 5 seconds instead of 3 seconds – it hits different! Try it! You have lots of different ways you can play around with the same workout, whilst easily being able to measure your progress.

Points to remember:

1. **FIND YOUR FEET** – Remember, they are your foundation.

2. **USE YOUR CORE** – The last exercise in the warm up (foam roller quadruped shoulder taps) should remind you of that feeling, so you can carry that with you throughout the main body of the workout.

3. **SLOWER EQUALS CONTROL** – If you're wobbling, slow it down, you've got this!

STRENGTH WITH EQUIPMENT – BEGINNER

Now we are ready to work with equipment. We are still focusing on moving well, especially now that we're adding load. Err on the side of caution with the weight you use – if every repetition feels easy, you have gone too light, if it feels heavy in the first few reps, you have gone too heavy. When the last one or two reps are a challenge, you have chosen the right weight.

WARM UP	MAIN WORKOUT	COOL DOWN
— Walk out (see page 145): 5 repetitions — Adductor rockback with rotation (see page 73): 3 repetitions each side — Foam roller deadbug (see page 141): 5 repetitions each side	— Goblet squat (see page 99): 2–3 sets of 8–10 repetitions — Romanian deadlift (see page 142): 2–3 sets of 8–10 repetitions — Bent leg ring row (see page 142): 2–3 sets of 8–10 repetitions — Single arm floor press (see page 143): 2-3 sets of 6-8 repetitions each side	— World's greatest stretch (see page 75): 3 repetitions each side — Scorpions with pec stretch (see page 138): 3 repetitions each side

To begin with, you could start with two sets in the main part of the workout. Once that feels comfortable, you can add a third set. As that starts to feel good, you could try two of the exercises back to back as a 'superset'. You have lots of different ways you can play around with the same workout, whilst easily being able to measure your progress.

STRENGTH WITH EQUIPMENT – INTERMEDIATE

WARM UP	MAIN WORKOUT	COOL DOWN
— Walk out (see page 145): 5 repetitions — Adductor rockback with rotation (see page 73): 3 repetitions each side — Foam roller deadbug (see page 141): 5 repetitions each side	— Offset goblet squat (see page 143): 2–3 sets of 8–10 repetitions — Single leg Romanian deadlift (see page 144): 2–3 sets of 6–8 repetitions on each leg — Straight leg ring row (see page 144): 2–3 sets of 8–10 repetitions — Floor press (see page 145): 2-3 sets of 8 repetitions	— World's greatest stretch (see page 75): 3 repetitions each side — Scorpions with pec stretch (see page 138): 3 repetitions each side

To begin with, you could start with two sets of the main workout. Once that feels comfortable, you can add a third set. As that starts to feel good, you could try two of the exercises back to back as a 'superset'. Or you could play around with the tempo at which you execute the movement – lowering down into an offset goblet squat for 3 seconds, then pausing in the bottom position for 2 seconds instead of coming straight back up will test you! Two seconds never felt so long! You have lots of different ways you can play around with the same workout, whilst easily being able to measure your progress.

Points to remember:

— Use a weight that makes the last one or two repetitions feel like work. If the last two reps feel easy, you've gone too light; if you didn't make it to the last two reps, you've gone too heavy.

— Video yourself doing the movement: a side-on or front-on diagonal view is usually pretty good to see most things. Sometimes how it looks and how it feels are two different things, so watching it back is really useful.

CARDIOVASCULAR FITNESS SESSION – BEGINNER

WARM UP	MAIN WORKOUT	COOL DOWN
— Walk out (see page 145): 5 repetitions — Adductor rockback with rotation (see page 73): 3 repetitions each side — Foam roller deadbug (see page 141): 5 repetitions each side	— **WEEK 1:** walk for 4 minutes, jog for 1 minute x 4 repetitions — **WEEK 2:** walk for 3 minutes, jog for 2 minutes x 4 repetitions — **WEEK 3:** walk for 2 minutes, jog for 3 minutes x 4 repetitions — **WEEK 4:** walk for 1 minute, jog for 4 minutes x 4 repetitions — **WEEK 5:** jog for 16–20 minutes	— World's greatest stretch (see page 75): 3 repetitions each side — Scorpions with pec stretch (see page 138): 3 repetitions each side

CARDIOVASCULAR FITNESS
SESSION – INTERMEDIATE

WARM UP	MAIN WORKOUT	COOL DOWN
— Walk out (see page 145): 5 repetitions — Adductor rockback with rotation (see page 73): 3 repetitions each side — Foam roller deadbug (see page 141) 5 repetitions each side	— **WEEK 1** = 20 minute run (jog for 4 minutes @ RPE 4-5, run for 1 minute @ RPE 6): x 4 — **WEEK 2** = 20 minute run (jog for 3 minutes @ RPE 4-5, run for 1 minute @ RPE 6): x 5 — **WEEK 3** = 18 minute run (jog for 2 minutes @ RPE 4-5, run for 1 minute @ RPE 6): x 6 — **WEEK 4** = 20 minute run (jog for 3 minutes @ RPE 4-5, run for 1 minute @ RPE 7): x 5 — **WEEK 5** = 18 minute run (jog for 2 minutes @ RPE 4-5, run for 1 minute @ RPE 7): x 6	— World's greatest stretch (see page 75) — Scorpions with pec stretch (see page 138)

And that concludes our strength and cardiovascular fitness programmes. Give them a try and see how you feel. A lot of the movements will feel new and so a little strange. Each time you do them they will feel more familiar. There is absolutely no rush with this – take it at your own pace and enjoy it.

EXERCISES EXPLAINED

KNEELING HIP HINGE

SET UP: Start by kneeling on the floor with your hands by your ears. Lift your bottom away from your heels so you are in a straight line from your knees to your head in a tall kneeling position.

1. Take a bow by letting your hips move backwards and your chest fall towards the floor, keeping your hands by your ears the whole time (this will help to prevent your back from rounding).

2. Return to the start position.

KNEELING PLANK ROW

SET UP: Set yourself up on all fours so your hands are underneath your shoulders and your knees are underneath your hips. Walk your hands forward so that your hips lower a little and there is a diagonal line running through your knees, hips, shoulders and all the way up to your head.

1. Lift your left hand off the floor, drawing your left elbow past your waist.

2. Return your left hand to the ground.

3. Lift your right hand off the floor, drawing your right elbow past your waist.

4. Return your right hand to the ground.

The key here is for your hips to remain static throughout the exercise and not move from side to side – this is very similar to the quadruped work we did with the foam roller.

ECCENTRIC PUSH UP

SET UP: Lie down on your front with your hands comfortably either side of your head, as if you were lying in bed. Place your hands where your elbows were, this is your hand position. Keeping your hands there, slowly come up onto your knees, or into a top plank position any way you can.

1. Keeping your whole body in a straight line, lower your body all the way down to the floor as slowly as possible.

2. Come back up to the start position any way you can.

The key here is that your whole body travels in a straight line. If you film yourself doing this, watch that your head doesn't jut forward or your hips sag too low – this takes practice, but you will get there.

SCORPIONS WITH PEC STRETCH

SET UP: Lie down on your front with your arms out to the sides.

1. Leading with your heel, take your right foot behind you, aiming for your left elbow so that your leg arcs diagonally behind you.

2. Lift your right arm up and reach towards the ceiling.

3. Return to the start position.

4. Take your left foot behind you, aiming for your right elbow so that your leg arcs diagonally behind you.

5. Lift your left arm up and reach towards the ceiling.

TEMPO GLUTE BRIDGE

SET UP: Lie down on your back with your legs bent and your feet flat on the floor, with your hands down by your sides.

1. Keep your feet firmly planted on the ground, take a deep inhale, and as you exhale, slowly lift your hips up towards the ceiling.

2. Inhale again, then slowly lower back down.

BULGARIAN SPLIT SQUAT

SET UP: Stand a few feet in front of a bench, facing away from it.

1. Place your left foot on top of the bench behind you; your right foot should still be facing forward with three points of contact with the ground.

2. Slowly sink your left knee towards the ground, keeping your chest nice and upright.

3. Slowly return to standing.

4. Repeat, placing your right foot on the bench and lowering your right knee towards the ground.

5. Slowly return to standing.

It's OK for there to be a slight forward lean in your upper body, but if you were doing this facing the mirror you should still be able to see the pocket of your t-shirt (imagine one if there is no pocket).

If you don't have a bench available or you feel this really challenges your balance, you could use something lower than a bench, like a yoga block or small stool.

HIGH PLANK ROW

SET UP: Set yourself up in a top plank position with your arms straight and your hands underneath your shoulders; your whole body should be in a straight line.

1. Lift your left hand off the floor, drawing your left elbow past your waist.

2. Return it to the ground.

3. Lift your right hand off the floor, bending your right elbow past your waist.

4. Return it to the ground.

The key here is for the hips not to move from side to side throughout the movement. Taking your feet wider will give you more of a stable base in this exercise. This is very similar to the quadruped work we did with the foam roller.

FOAM ROLLER DEADBUG

SET UP: You will need a foam roller for this. Lie on your back with your hips and knees both bent to 90 degrees. Place one end of the foam roller above your knee on your left thigh, and support the other end in place with your right arm, ensuring your arm is kept straight (the foam roller should be placed just below your wrist). Straighten your left arm towards the ceiling to line it up with the right arm

1. Keeping downward pressure with your arm on the foam roller throughout, take a deep breath in, then, as you exhale, slowly straighten your right leg towards the ground and straighten your left arm behind you at the same time (don't let your foot or hand touch the ground as you straighten them, allow them to hover an inch above the ground).

2. Inhale and return the right leg and left arm back to the start position.

3. Repeat the same on the other side, this time, with the foam roller above your knee on your right thigh supported by your left arm.

ROMANIAN DEADLIFT

SET UP: Stand with your feet hip-width apart, holding dumbbells in each hand in front of your thighs. Squeeze your shoulder blades together and down as if you are placing them in your back pockets.

1. With a soft bend in the knees, shift your hips backwards (your shoulder blades should still be squeezed together and down), allowing the dumbbells to shave down your thighs to just past your knees.

2. Return to start position.

Doing the kneeling hip hinge exercise on page 136 just before this as movement preparation is really useful as it mimics what your body needs to do in this exercise.

BENT LEG RING ROW

SET UP: Set a pair of gymnastic rings or a TRX at hip height. Placing your hands on the rings, position yourself below the rings with your legs bent and your body parallel to the floor.

1. With both palms facing one another on the rings, lift your chest towards the rings by drawing your elbows back past your waist.

2. Slowly lower back down.

SINGLE ARM FLOOR PRESS

SET UP: Lie on your back with your legs bent and feet on the floor. Hold a dumbbell in your left hand extended towards the ceiling; your right arm can be down by your side.

1. Take a deep breath in and slowly lower your left elbow towards the ground, keeping your forearm perpendicular to the floor and the angle of your elbow lower than your shoulder.

2. Exhale and return your arm to start position. Repeat on the other side.

OFFSET GOBLET SQUAT

SET UP: Hold a dumbbell in your left hand, just in front of your shoulder. Stand tall with your feet slightly wider than hip-width apart and slightly turned out to create a little extra space through your hips. Ensure both feet are in full contact with the ground keeping those three points of contact.

1. Letting your knees and hips flex at the same time, slowly lower your hips back and down into a squat.

2. Stand back up, keeping those three points of contact with the ground throughout.

3. Repeat holding the dumbbell in your right hand.

SINGLE LEG ROMANIAN DEADLIFT

SET UP: Stand with your feet hip-width apart, holding dumbbells in each hand in front of your thighs. Squeeze your shoulder blades together and down as if you are placing them in your back pockets.

1. Starting by standing on your right leg only, with a soft bend in your right knee. Shift your hips backwards, letting the left leg travel behind you (your shoulder blades should still be squeezed together and down) and keeping the dumbbells close to your body until you are just past the knee.

2. Return to start position.

If you find this challenging, try the single leg version without weight, or try the same single leg movement with your hands by your ears.

STRAIGHT LEG RING ROW

SET UP: Set a pair of gymnastic rings or a TRX at hip height. Placing your hands on the rings, position yourself below the rings with your legs straight and your body parallel to the floor.

1. With both palms facing one another on the rings, lift your chest towards the rings by drawing your elbows back past your waist.

2. Slowly lower back down.

The more parallel you are to the ground, the more challenging this is.

FLOOR PRESS

SET UP: Lie on your back with your legs bent and your feet on the floor. Hold a dumbbell in each hand, with your arms extended towards the ceiling.

1. Take a deep breath in and slowly lower your elbows towards the ground, keeping your forearms perpendicular to the floor and the angle of your elbows lower than your shoulders.

2. Exhale and return to the start position.

WALKOUT

SET UP: Stand with your feet underneath your hips.

1. With a soft bend in the knees, slowly roll your body down to place your hands on the floor, then slowly walk your hands out into a top plank.

2. Return to start position, by walking the hands back and slowly curling back up again to standing.

FOAM ROLLER QUADRUPED SHOULDER TAPS

SET UP: You will need a foam roller, water bottle or anything cylindrical. Position yourself on all fours, then place the roller horizontally across your lower back.

1. Lift your knees one inch off the ground and focus on keeping the roller on your back.

2. Touch your left shoulder with your right hand, and place it back on the ground. Then touch your right shoulder with your left hand, and place it back down. Continue touching the opposite shoulder with the opposite hand, without the foam roller falling off your back.

CHAPTER 10

KEEP IT GOING

OK, so I have lured you into the world of fitness. Hopefully I have soothed your fears by showing you that you are already doing some of the basics and a little tweak here and there will just upgrade your practice and get you embracing movement more. Now I've warmed you up with the big four – showing you their individual magnificence and how together they are an absolute force – you may feel more encouraged to start there, to fold the exercises I laid out into your daily routine. However, what happens when – and it will come – one day you're just not feeling it. You see, I can lay all of the above on a plate for you, but I have to make sure that the damn thing is going to work for you, and for your life. One size most definitely does not fit all. You are so unique and fabulous that you have to run your own party for this show to work. So, let's see what that looks like.

HOW IT ALL FITS

TIME

If you're not a morning person, then there's a high chance that a 7am class is not going to work for you. Instead, think about scheduling lunch hour or evening sessions. Always make sure that what you choose fits into your life, and suits how your world operates. Don't commit to something you're not suited to.

YES OR NO

It's a simple question – do you like it? So many 'shoulds' fly around with exercise. If running makes you cry every step of the way and makes you recite 'this is shit' on repeat, maybe it's not for you. Although I challenge you to expand your knowledge on what constitutes exercise. If you have boxed yourself into the idea that fitness is just beasting it in the gym or taking your pins for a spin, then a: I'm disappointed (just kidding, but sort of not) and b: get ready because there is a whole world out there that has your name on it, that says, 'exercise you actually like, this way!'

LIFE

My friend and fellow coach Allison Tenney always asks, 'Can you still make it work when life gets "lifey"?' She understands how life can throw relentless curve balls at us, and even with the best intentions, something has to give. A common example of this is when a client of mine has three sessions a week planned in. Life gets, yep, lifey and they just manage to squeeze one full session in. Enthusiastically, they promise to make up for the missed sessions the following week and do four and a half sessions instead of the three programmed. No, just no. Let's look at why some of the sessions were missed and see how we can adapt the following week to make them work. And maybe we don't. Maybe two sessions *is* what works. Great, let's roll with that!

PERSISTENCE

OK, so maybe you don't love it because you don't feel like you're good at it yet. I'm not beating the do-whatever-it-takes drum but, to get better at something, you need to do it more, even when it feels like it sucks. (May I present to you the four question review on page 43? You're welcome!) When I make a commitment to get better at something, particularly when it comes to movement, I give myself twelve weeks. Twelve weeks of showing up, even when progress feels slow. I tell myself twelve weeks is a good amount of time to evaluate progress.

NON-NEGOTIABLE

Not to be confused with how can I get fit by doing nothing. But what is your non-negotiable – your minimum effective dose – to stay on a committed path. You are committed, aren't you? I mean, we've made it this far. I'll even let you call me 'Jos' (it's 'Joslyn' to strangers). We're on one-syllable terms now. The previous techniques I've showed you are really helpful here. Can you commit to switching off your phone 30 minutes before bed, at least three times a week? Seven nights would be great, but let's make three your minimum effective dose, and how about getting a good amount of hours in. Can you take five deep breaths in the morning when you wake up? You know, before you pick up your phone. Taking the time to pause for five breaths three times a day would be epic, but let's work to make it that when you wake up, you achieve your minimum effective dose. You see where I'm going here? You may have an idea in your head of what would be your ideal, but you also need to decide what you are not going to shift on.

HABIT STACKING

In James Clear's book *Atomic Habits*, he talks about the concept of habit stacking. When you are trying to build a new habit into your life, build it into something you already do regularly. Adding that breathwork as soon as you wake up is easy to make happen every day, right? Because you always – thankfully – wake up each day. So the very next thing you can do is take those five breaths. You are 'stacking' your new focused breathing habit onto your current habit of waking up. In the book, Clear breaks down all the steps it takes to go to the gym, including packing your bag the night before, leaving the house in enough time to get there, the journey there, and then stepping inside the gym. Quite a few steps, right? Except, he suggests just packing your bag the night before, and doing that for a few days. Then you do your journey to the gym, repeating that for a few days. Then you finally step inside the gym, except when you get there you stay for just five minutes. Weird, right? But it all makes sense. How often have you been motivated to do something and you haven't fully thought through all the steps that get you there? Then you can't find your keys, or your ticket or your trainers or whatever you need. I hold both my hands up to this! The method that Clear suggests makes absolute sense. If we don't create the habit or establish the routine around it, our own enthusiasm to just get going can get in the way. Start with baby steps, there's no rush.

VARIETY AND INTENSITY

One of the ways to keep your new movement plan fresh is to add a bit of variety. So now that we have the basics, how do you change things up or add intensity? Variety doesn't mean doing a completely new exercise – a simple change in stance, going from both legs (bilateral) to one leg (unilateral), grip position or positioning in general, or changing equipment all add a new stimulus.

In the fitness world, intensity can often be interpreted as sweating more. But intensity is not just a measure of how much you sweat. Intensity can be any of the following:

LOAD – increase or decrease the weight

SUPERSETS – doing two exercises back to back

TEMPO – change the time under tension

REST PERIOD – reduce the amount of rest in between sets

VOLUME – increase the number of sets or repetitions

Take any exercise and increase the weight, take longer to do the movement, give yourself less rest in between movements, or more of the movement and add intensity. If we want to go deeper on that idea, let's include the intensity of life. What would happen to the same exercise session if you'd had little sleep the night before, or work was incredibly stressful? Would it be more intense? Yep! And that's OK. Awareness is key. Exercise is a stress on the body. If you are tired and already stressed, you will feel it. This is where rate of perceived exertion discussed on page 112 comes in handy – you work to the level your body can handle. An exercise that feels like a comfortable 5 on a good day, may feel like a 7 when you are short on sleep or feeling highly stressed.

For women, we can also consider the menstrual cycle as a determinant of the level of intensity at different stages across the month. The follicular phase (the first day of your period until ovulation – roughly days 1–14) lends itself to a higher work rate, increased strength and recovery; and the luteal phase (from ovulation to just before your period) lends itself to a lower work rate and reduced recovery. Again, this is influenced by recovery in general: sleep, food, hydration, stress levels.

TRACKING

OK, I realise I've said this about a few things so far, but if there is another thing I want you to take away with you, it's tracking. The more information you have about yourself, for yourself, the better able you are to make decisions about your health. It's also a great motivator to see how far you've come and encourage you to keep going.

If you feel it matters, write it down. Your training, your sleep, your food, your water intake, your time out to breathe. You can do that any way you want – on paper, on your phone, on a paper towel – whatever works best for you. But, and this is a big but, if tracking stresses you in any way (this is a big one when it comes to food), do the following: keep it simple, a mark out of 10 will suffice, rather than going any deeper on detail; or stop tracking if you feel it is becoming an unhealthy obsession. In the same way that people take time out from, or limit, their social media intake, I would suggest doing the same for tracking.

MEASURING AND GETTING RESULTS

It's simple: consistency is what will get you there, my darlings! Consistency in training. Consistency in your tracking. Consistency in putting yourself first. Sing it with me – CON – SIST – EN – CY.

In the beginning, it's likely that with just a little consistency, you will start to see results – more energy, more confidence in the movements, that bossy feeling you get when you are doing something good for your body. As long as you are continuing to see results, keep going. Remember those boring things like sleep and breathing that light your world on fire. Doing the same thing and still getting results is the name of the game!

GOING FURTHER

You can honestly take this where you want to. You understand ALL the pieces of the puzzle now. Want to work your tail off? You better have a hot recovery plan. Want to build strength? Don't short-change yourself and skip on mobility. Want to run a race for charity? Build that cardiac output, power up with some strength work and don't slack on recovery.

FIND YOUR PEOPLE

You don't have to do this alone. I mean, you still have to show up for you, because nobody else is going to do the work for you, but you're not alone. It's always better when you find your people, who feel the exact same way about this whole movement thing as you do – a little apprehensive, a little excited, and with a desire to keep this damn thing going.

Some of my favourite approaches to a commitment to movement were developed by those who didn't see a space for themselves in fitness.

Brothers Tayler and Koen Prince-Fraser set up a running club called Last Pick Athletics Club (LPAC). Yep, if you got picked last in PE, guess what – you have found your people! My friend Cory Wharton-Malcolm set up a running crew called Track Mafia and cushioned the 'boredom' of running by creating a community around it. The group would go for coffee beforehand and food after, therefore building their meets around life activities with a snippet of training in between. My friend Dora Atim set up Ultra Black Running, a safe space for black wxmen, girls and gender non-conforming folk to explore the world of trail running. My friend Jonelle

Lewis taught yoga to people without yoga mats in public spaces like libraries, teaching that you didn't need nice leggings, candles and zen studios to build your yoga practice, making it accessible to all! The essence of them all is community, and the creation of something that didn't exist for that community. It may be that a particular community you are interested in joining isn't quite for you. You may not see people like you there, or the vibe could be off. You know what to do then – start your own damn thing! I don't care if you don't have experience, get some friends together and just do it. What's to stop you grabbing a few friends and kicking a ball around in a park, or going for a run, or setting up your own team? If you were never 'sporty' because you felt different, then find your people and start. Because what we do know is that we all need to move. And you never know where you can take it either. Let's just dream a little. What if you started this movement thing, got a few friends involved, decided to apply some of the basics that we have covered, and got pretty good? Now, I'm not saying the Olympics are in sight because that's a lifelong endeavour, but our bodies are amazing; finding out where you can take yours is a beautiful journey of the body and mind.

CONCLUSION

So that's it. All my feels on how to move it. I don't yet know anyone who has regretted adding more movement into their life, and I have witnessed many lives it has completely changed. But we have become so transfixed on what fitness means, concerning ourselves with the perception of it rather than what the reality is for us. Our reality. Our version of movement. For us. It's pretty special when we find it.

Whatever 'sporty' thing you decide to do, remember, YOU HAVE GOT THIS! You know all the things, and you already do a lot of them. You have a body, so you are an athlete, remember! In case you ever forget, here's a quick check in:

1. **STAY POSITIVE** – Reframe those nagging thoughts that are telling you you're not capable of doing that run or lifting that weight. As Henry Ford famously said, 'Whether you think you can or think you can't, you're right.' If you are having a bad day or feeling demotivated, read through chapter 1 and be amazed by the power of the mind. Yes, yours.

2. **START WITH THE BASICS** – That you already do. Can you improve the quality of your sleep? Breathe a bit deeper? Move around a little

more? Great, you've already made the first step, and the most important thing is just to start.

3. **SET AN INTENTION FOR YOUR GOAL** – What steps do you need to take to get there? A play around with mobility? The bodyweight beginner programme? But don't get stuck in the planning stage – take messy action, dive in and learn as you go.

4. **NOTE IT DOWN** – Reviewing any action you take, no matter how small, with a view to any improvements that could be made, will help you to navigate your training journeys better. And the simplest way to stay motivated is to track your progress.

5. **FIND THE FUN** – What would you love to do that you never felt 'sporty' enough to do? Make an enquiry. Book it. Bring a friend.

If you made it all the way here, thank you for committing to moving better; it means the world to me and you won't regret a moment of it.

everyday resources

Here's some further resources to keep you going.

PODCASTS
Fitness Unfiltered
Trained by Nike

APPS
Nike Training Club
Headspace
Moody Month

PEOPLE
Cory Wharton-Malcolm - @trackmafia
Dora Atim - @ultrablackrunning
Emma Hackett – www.limitlesscoaching.co.uk
Katie Page – www.mindtrainingforsport.co.uk
Jonelle Lewis – www.jonellelewis.com

BOOKS
James Clear, *Atomic Habits* (2018)

acKNOWLedGeMeNts

This was my first foray into writing a book so to say I did it not knowing what the hell I was doing is an understatement. So, my first thank you is to the person who got me into this mess, Lemara Lindsay-Prince, commissioning editor for #Merky Books. Lemara, I cannot state enough that I could not have done this without you, your skills of persuasion are second to none, and you moved heaven and earth for me even when the deadlines were long gone! You made this whole experience a joy and always knew exactly what to say and when to say it. I am forever grateful that you got me through and I have gained a lifelong friend. To Mica Murphy, Design Lead at Penguin, thank you so very much for bringing what is so important to me, to life, in your illustrations for the book. You are incredible, thank you. Thank you #Merky Books for this incredible 'How to' series, what an honour to be part of such an incredible project.

To my own mentors, my husband BJ Rule, CJ Swaby, Andrew Marshall and Robbie Peters, not sure you'll ever understand how much you have influenced my work - to watch you from near and afar, you taught me about the kind of coach I wanted to be and still do. I am forever grateful. Thank you.

To my 'Be The Change' crew, thank you for letting me be vulnerable in this tough year - you got me through it more than you know, and you inspire me daily, it takes my breath away.

To Nita and Neha for getting me through the wobbles, you sense what I need before I even know myself and hit me with a hard dose of reality when I'm being annoying. I love you both with my whole heart. Courts, you have never not been there, the timeliness and grace of your checking in, or not, is perfection. Thank you.

To BJ, no matter what I decide to do, you never question it, you just support me from start to finish. You don't complete me, you let me be me, there is nothing more I need. Thank you and I love you. To Bjorn and Max, thank you for choosing me, you teach me every day about life and love and wrestling, I love you so very much.

NOTES

NOTES

NOTES

NOTES

NOTES

NOTES

NOTES

NOTES

NOTES

NOTES

NOTES

UNLOCK YOUR POTENTIAL WITH THE *HOW TO* SERIES

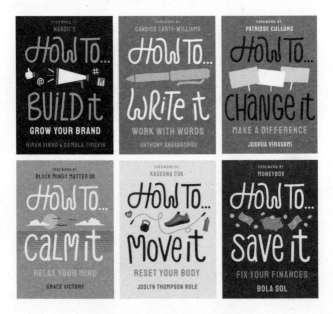

AVAILABLE NOW

FOLLOW @MERKYBOOKS FOR NEWS ON THE NEXT *HOW TO* RELEASES ...